STO

STROKE

STROKE

THE NEW HOPE
AND
THE NEW HELP

DR. ARTHUR S. FREESE

Random House 🏠 New York

Published in the United States by Random House, Inc., New York, and
simultaneously in Canada by Random House of Canada Limited, Toronto.

Library of Congress Cataloging in Publication Data
Freese, Arthur S
Stroke: the new hope and the new help.
Bibliography: p.
Includes index.
I. Cerebrovascular disease. I. Title.
RC388.5.F73   616.8'1   80–5415
ISBN 0–394–50179–9

Manufactured in the United States of America
24689753
First Edition

This book is dedicated to
the victims of stroke and their families,
and to those in the field of rehabilitation
who have long struggled to aid and educate
both the public and the members of the medical profession
alike about the new promise and help for stroke victims

ACKNOWLEDGMENTS

In a very real sense this book owes its being to the many who have suffered the tragedy of stroke, and to their families—as well as to all those professionals who have devoted so much of their lives to the struggle against it. Obviously I cannot list by name all those who have contributed to this book; I hope they will all accept my thanks without specific mention. However, certain individuals and organizations do stand out:

Dr. James C. Folsom, Director of ICD Rehabilitation and Research Center; Dr. Joseph Brudny, Director ICD Sensory Feedback Therapy Unit; the National Easter Seal Society; the American Heart Association and its Science Information Chief, Howard L. Lewis; the Society for Neuroscience and its Public Relations Consultants, Estelle and Eugene Kone; the National Institute of Neurological and Communicative Disorders and Stroke; the National Heart, Lung, and Blood Institute; Robert B. O'Connell, Spcl. Asst. to the Asst. Secy. of our Dept. of Health and Human Services (formerly Health, Education and Welfare).

Very special appreciation and thanks to my very talented editor, Robert D. Loomis; along with an appreciation of my long-suffering wife, Ruth.

CONTENTS

INTRODUCTION

It is important to know that the world of stroke has recently been turned upside down by the development of a whole new dimension —one that has suddenly made the future bright with a variety of promises and hopes. But, tragically, many still regard stroke as it was once looked upon in our unhappy, and fortunately now obsolete, medical past. Those old, mistaken concepts still persist— among them the belief that a stroke victim has no alternative but to wait (usually in a wheelchair or bed) for the second and eventually the third and fatal episode to strike mysteriously and at random.

Now, for the first time in man's history, there are actually means of *preventing* strokes. These include the simple act of taking a tiny white pill a few times a day, or of merely becoming familiar with the risk factors (including one, for example, that makes some women twenty times as susceptible as others doing the same thing) and then just avoiding them. And for those unfortunates who have already suffered this tragic disease there are new methods for recovery which they and their families should know about—help that is now available even to those who were stricken several years ago and more.

Stroke, in fact, threatens us all. It afflicts both sexes, from the infant in the crib to the very old, although it does have certain favorites. It has stricken our Presidents—from John Quincy Adams to Franklin Delano Roosevelt and Dwight D. Eisenhower (and his wife Mamie)—and such well-known figures as Walt Whitman and Cornelia Otis Skinner. And almost all of us can recall a relative or friend, a co-worker or neighbor who has suffered a stroke.

Because it inevitably strikes so close to all our homes, it is vital to learn more about this dread disease. With knowledge we can protect ourselves, our stricken family members and friends, from the worst effects of stroke—and even more important, we can learn how to *prevent* it. So damaging is a stroke to those close to the victims that one nationally known expert—Dr. James C. Folsom, director of ICD Rehabilitation and Research Center and formerly head of Rehabilitation Medicine for the entire Veterans Administration—feels strongly that "the basic problem of stroke is the effect it has on the family—everything else, no matter what, ends up being the residual of this effect." What this damage is and how to deal with it will also be covered in our book.

This image of stroke that persists from out of the past is one of complete helplessness in the face of an unpredictable, unexpected disaster, striking at random without reason or warning. But now we know that this is not only wrong but self-destructive, for believing this keeps victims and families from the very hope that, with modern medical expertise, makes possible both recovery and a return to the good life once more.

To correct such damaging misunderstandings is in good part what this book is all about: here is what stroke really is and who is in danger of it; how it can be prevented; and how the majority of its victims can be restored to a good quality of life, can be made functioning human beings once more. This can't be overemphasized, for too many people are cheated even today of a decent life after suffering their strokes simply because much of the medical profession has failed to keep abreast with the latest findings.

As a result, the victim and his family alone can ensure the best medical care by learning what help is available and where, and by insisting that a worthwhile productive life is the right of every stroke victim today. Far too often, physicians tend to write off the stroke sufferer, feeling that if the patient doesn't respond or recover in a matter of a few months after the incident, then his case is hopeless. Doctors often take a "Well, you just have to accept it" attitude without providing their patients with access to the vast array of specialized and skilled medical help actually available today.

Should this statement seem extreme, let us listen to two leading stroke experts. Dr. Oscar M. Reinmuth, professor of neurology at the University of Pittsburgh, warns of the large number of physicians who, even today, are unaware of the skilled help available to stroke patients. The result, in his words, is "the abysmal lack of interest in such matters as adequate diagnoses, treatment, and rehabilitation that are the rule rather than the exception throughout much of our land." And Dr. Joseph Brudny, a New York University professor of rehabilitation medicine and director of ICD Sensory Feedback Therapy Unit, is dismayed by the failure of our medical system to really concern itself with these sufferers: "Stroke is the orphan of American medicine—and this has to change because younger and younger people are being afflicted. The old idea that stroke was part of the natural process of dying—you died in two installments, first you had the stroke and then you died—just isn't true any more!"

The whole aim of this book is to give readers the tools and the information they may need to secure proper medical care and rehabilitation should this disease strike. Above all else, this information will give readers an awareness of why no stroke victim should ever give up, for there are new and highly successful techniques which experts can now utilize to help restore the use of arms and legs to victims whose strokes have robbed them of the use of these limbs, even though this may have happened many years before.

This, then, is a book of hope and promise to light up a dark corner of disease, one which afflicts millions of Americans. Here is what you need to know to understand the disorder, and either to prevent it or to ensure proper medical care and help to secure a good quality of functioning life should this disease strike.

In the use of the personal pronoun in this book, the "he" will be used chiefly, since men are stricken far more often than women. However, it should be recognized that this is done because it is the simpler way—and read it as referring to either man or woman.

I

THE BASICS OF STROKE

1

THE STORY OF STROKE

The Terms Doctors Use; the Statistics; the Victims, Their Ages and Sexes; the New Hope

Whether it's called stroke or apoplexy, as it was in the past, this disease has long carried with it an aura of mystery and finality that terrifies mankind. Which is not surprising, for until our own generation this disease seemingly struck its victims without warning, leaving them hopelessly paralyzed and also often incapable of speech and other means of communication. Forsaken by a helpless medical profession, these sufferers were relegated to wheelchair or bed, to back bedroom or nursing home, where they awaited succeeding strokes which would increasingly incapacitate them until a final one proved fatal.

Since its causes were not understood, this disease was regarded as a sort of natural concomitant of old age, even though until very recently man's life span was quite short. The average life span of the ancient Greeks and Romans was around twenty-seven or twenty-eight years—and in medieval England this had only increased to thirty-two. Our own first national census, in 1790, revealed that fewer than one in five Americans reached the Biblical three score and ten years—whereas today more than four out of five of us can anticipate living beyond this age.

If stroke were truly only a disease of old age there would have been very few instances of it until relatively recent times, since there were simply not enough older people around. But as Dr. Oscar M. Reinmuth, University of Pittsburgh stroke expert, explains, this disease strikes "anyone, from the newborn, the infant, the youth, and the young adult to even you and me in the years of our greatest usefulness to family and society."

Hippocrates, the father of medicine over two thousand years ago, wrote: "It is impossible to remove [cure] a strong attack of apoplexy, and not easy to remove [cure] a weak attack." This bleak medical view of stroke continued until barely a generation ago but has now certainly been turned completely around. Of course, a severe massive attack such as that suffered by President Franklin Roosevelt still proves fatal, but we can now prevent and even, on occasion, cure stroke, which means that its victims can be returned to a life whose quality is once more worthwhile and satisfying.

To start to learn about this problem and how to protect ourselves, we must be familiar with the words and the terms used.

The Terms Doctors Use

The oldest term applied to this disease—and one that is only rarely heard anymore—is the one Hippocrates used, *apoplexy.* The most widely used name for this disease is surely *stroke*—and it implies the element of suddennesss (to strike) that seems so characteristic of the problem. A stroke is actually a sudden loss of brain (cerebral) function, which results from an interference with the normal blood supply to that organ (later we'll discuss the many causes in detail).

Physicians and other scientists working in this field often term strokes *cerebrovascular accidents* (CVAs for short). This is both more accurate and more descriptive, for "cerebro" refers to the brain and "vascular" to the blood vessels, while the accident part emphasizes the abrupt nature of the loss of cerebral function.

Physicians also use another word—*hemiplegia*—almost synonymously with stroke or CVA. This is actually a misnomer ("hemi" means half and "plegia" paralysis), for while strokes almost always affect half the body, only very rarely is there truly a total paralysis or loss of function; rather, there is a weakness or muscle spasm (again, details will come later).

You should also be familiar with the terms *cerebral infarct* or *infarction.* An infarct is an area of damaged, dying or dead tissue, usually due to the loss of its blood supply. While by infarction may be meant the process leading to the formation of an infarct, doctors often also use the term cerebral infarction to mean an infarct—and both these terms are used interchangeably with stroke or CVA. (For further explanation of terms, see Chapter 3.)

How Common Is Stroke and What Does It Cost Us?

The latest statistics of our National Institute of Neurological and Communicative Disorders and Stroke (NINCDS) reveal that there are about 2.5 million disabled stroke survivors in this country. Experts estimate that some 600,000 Americans are stricken afresh every year and that roughly 40 percent of these die. In fact, CVA ranks third among our leading causes of death and is exceeded only by heart disease and cancer. In short, strokes incapacitate far more people than they kill, and are probably the leading cause of long-term disability in the United States.

NINCDS experts admit that "no detailed estimates of the monetary losses sustained by stroke victims can be made with available data." Opinions of the total annual economic toll this disease takes do vary; one figure for the cost of caring for stroke victims runs to $12.5 billion. But this does not really cover the true toll of this disease, as NINCDS experts emphasize: "Lives are stunted or for all practical purposes ended; families are disrupted or impoverished for months or years; and valuable contributors are lost to society."

It is now believed that six out of every hundred persons will suffer a stroke sometime in his or her lifetime. However, the stroke picture is not entirely clear at this time; for one thing, there has been evidence that both the incidence of CVAs and the death rate have been dropping during the last thirty to fifty years. This trend has not been clear-cut, because doctors themselves confuse the picture with diagnostic inaccuracies and their following of current medical fashions in diagnoses. Then, too, there are changes in death-certification methods, and the like.

The city of Rochester, Minnesota, home of the Mayo Clinic, represents a unique situation which is virtually the dream of the epidemiologists (those experts who study the statistics of diseases, the factors involved in the frequency and distribution of disorders): in Rochester virtually all medical diagnoses—at the Mayo Clinic, at the hospitals and in the private offices of all but one or two private physicians—are recorded in an automated record-retrieval system. Moreover, many of these diagnoses are confirmed by autopsies, since these are performed on over half of those who die, something rare elsewhere in the United States. As a result there are near-total medical histories available for those local residents who have sought medical care during the past several decades.

Taking advantage of this unique situation, a team of Mayo Clinic epidemiologists headed by Dr. W. Michael Garroway recently reported on their study of the incidence of stroke in Rochester from 1945 to 1974. They found that for every one hundred first episodes of stroke which occurred during the years 1945 to 1949, there were only fifty-five new ones in the period 1970 to 1974. This drop in CVAs occurred in all age groups and both sexes, but the greatest reduction was found among those eighty years of age and older.

Experts do not accept this change at its full face value because there are some nagging questions remaining. For example, Dr. Jack P. Whisnant, chairman of the Mayo Clinic department of neurology and a member of this team, points out that the Rochester area is predominantly white, so the findings may not apply equally to blacks. An NINCDS poll of United States hospitals may also eventually show this decline—for blacks as well as for whites.

Questions, too, must be raised about the fact that over the last fifty years there has been a decline in stroke deaths: from 1968 to 1977 these stroke death rates dropped 32 percent. Experts raise the possibility that the mortality is declining not because the incidence rate has gone down but because there is improved medical care with less recurrences and a lowered fatality rate.

Along with such hopeful signs (perhaps due to the very preventive measures we will suggest later) there are problems as well. NINCDS experts point out that there are rapidly increasing numbers of Americans living longer today and reaching those very ages which are most at risk where stroke is concerned. And one cannot ignore the tragic data showing that stroke is still third among the causes of death. Furthermore, there are still many other unresolved questions and bizarre facts about this disorder.

The Stroke Belt and the Carolina-Cairo Connection: The World-Wide Geography of Stroke

Looking at the global picture, Dr. Joseph Brudny points out that "stroke is becoming the leading neurological disability throughout the world. We once thought that it just struck the more advanced countries of North America and Europe—but we now find it as prevalent or more so in South America and Central Africa, in India, Japan, and in China, where it is now the number-one killer." In fact, in Japan 500 of every 100,000 people die from stroke—as compared to only 146 per 100,000 in the United States.

Such great geographical differences in stroke morbidity (proportion of disease in a locality) and mortality have for many years been noted by epidemiologists. The current "stroke belt" concept can best be understood by looking at a map showing stroke death rates in the United States. There is a broad band of the highest rates running south from North Carolina, through South Carolina and Georgia, touching northern Florida and continuing into Alabama and Mississippi, and upward into Tennessee. There are also pockets of high CVA death rates in Texas and Oklahoma, and all the Hawaiian Islands. Wide differences are also seen in the causes involved. In Japan, for example, most fatal strokes result from hypertension (high blood pressure) and cerebral hemorrhage. But in the United States the chief cause is blockage of the cerebral arteries resulting from atherosclerosis (hardening of the arteries).

Dr. James F. Toole, professor of neurology at Wake Forest University, has been studying these stroke rates and finds wide variations even in such relatively small geographical areas as his own state of North Carolina. While the state's coastal plains suffer what is almost the highest death rate from stroke in the nation, its Blue Ridge mountain areas, less than two hundred miles away, enjoy some of our lowest stroke mortality rates. These statistics lead this expert to suspect that there may be "environmental, cultural or other geographically determined risk factors."

Dr. Toole feels that "many risk factors for stroke are not heredi-tary but are implanted during youth." This is shown, he points out, in the NI-HON-SAN study of Japanese stroke rates in three differ-ent communities: Hiroshima, a high-risk area (one with a high CVA mortality rate, such as the stroke belt); Honolulu, an inter-mediate-risk one; and San Francisco with low risk. The study shows that those Japanese who grew up in Hiroshima and later moved to Honolulu or San Francisco remained at high risk despite their move. But their children and grandchildren born in these American communities showed a decreased risk. In other words, the person who grows up in a high-risk area will continue to have a greater likelihood of stroke even if, as an adult, he moves to a low-risk section. Similarly, being raised in and moving from a low-risk community will not put a person in greater danger of a CVA should he, as an adult, move to a high-risk area. "This has . . . led to speculation that the risk factor may be dietary or cultural," Dr. Toole explains. "Alternatively, one might consider that the risk is related to altitude or water supply."

Differences in the minerals in the water people drink; the alti-tudes at which they live; their differing cultures, customs and foods; even the distances at which their homes are from the ocean —all these have been proposed as causes for the wide differences in stroke rates such as occur in North Carolina, in the stroke belt there and elsewhere. Dr. Toole sees a medical opportunity in the geography of the Nile River and the nature of the people who live alongside it—a means by which he can learn about the reasons for the stroke belt and North Carolina with its high stroke risk. He likes to call this project "the Carolina-Cairo Connection."

The neurologist points out that, unlike North Carolina, Egypt's Nile River area is surprisingly uniform. The people and their customs are unusually homogeneous, and they use the same water supply, the Nile itself. Moreover, the elevation along the river varies by less than three hundred feet. There are only two really significant differences along the Nile, from a stroke-rate point of view: distance from the Mediterranean and varying temperatures. Thus, if stroke rates are due to either of these factors, this Cairo study will prove it—and if not, then the Carolina differences can only be due to a now limited group of factors from which Dr. Toole would then hope to isolate the cause. Should these stroke-risk factors prove to be ones that can be altered by man (say, the minerals in drinking water), it is certainly not beyond the realm of possibility that the stroke belt itself may in the future become a thing of the past, and the terrible toll of stroke itself be reduced.

Who Suffer Strokes?

Strokes are obviously no respecters of persons, striking all ages and races, and both sexes. However, the disease does play favorites, striking certain groups most heavily and often for reasons which doctors still don't clearly understand. Stroke is a sexist disorder, for twice as many men as women suffer strokes—which may very likely be related to the higher incidence of hypertension and atherosclerosis in men. Perhaps, too, female hormones exert some protective influence here; this even led to some attempts in the past to prevent strokes in men by giving them female sex hormones, but the resulting feminization, with enlarged breasts and loss of sexual drive, pretty much stopped this. Young women also have a lower death rate than men from heart attacks—but after the menopause this rate increases sharply, although it never reaches the level of that of men.

Differences in morbidity and mortality rates from stroke between different racial groups, and even the same racial groups in different environments, have been noted. Black Americans are 50 percent more likely to have hypertension than whites, and this, as we shall see, is now a widely recognized and major factor in causing strokes. So it is not surprising to find that blacks suffer more strokes

—and more severe ones—as well as having them at a younger age. Perhaps lifestyle and diet, stress and familial tendencies all play some part.

Studies have been made of the cholesterol found in cerebral blood vessels obtained in autopsies of American blacks and whites, and of Nigerian Africans, all living in urban areas. The investigators found that Washington, D.C., blacks had more than three times as much cerebral vascular cholesterol as the Ibadan Nigerians, while Minneapolis whites were roughly in the middle. This would seem to be related to the greater severity and degree of cerebral atherosclerosis and stroke in American blacks.

While no age is free from stroke, people are not all evenly afflicted. The incidence of CVAs does rise steadily with increasing age, and the peak age period is generally considered to be the sixties. Only 20 percent of strokes occur before the age of sixty-five, and a long-term study of some thousand patients at the Cornell Division of New York's Bellevue Hospital found that only 8 percent of victims suffered their CVAs before the age of fifty. The American Heart Association reports that 1 out of 6 stroke deaths occur before the age of sixty-five. A particularly tragic side of the disease is that it strikes the newborn and even those still in the womb. In fact, a team of experts assembled by NINCDS and headed by Dr. Arnold P. Gold, a Columbia University professor of pediatric neurology, points out that it is believed that 5 percent of stroke patients admitted to our hospitals are below the age of twenty.

But the picture is changing now. As Dr. Brudny explains: "Today stroke is not uncommon in the forties and fifties, and I see stroke patients in the hospital in their late thirties. Too many young people are having strokes because we have a higher degree of stressful situations in our lives; there is an increased tendency for clotting in young women taking oral contraceptive medications; and there are three million head injuries each year, some of whom have strokes due to such trauma." The American Heart Association, too, finds that CVAs are striking younger people at an alarming rate.

What Effect Will a Stroke Have on One's Life?

This question looms large when such disorders strike. Perhaps the best way to answer is simply to look at some who have suffered strokes—individuals whose life work is so demanding that any loss or diminution of their powers would be quickly apparent.

First the extreme, and one of our country's most shocking experiences. On April 12, 1945, as World War II was winding down in Europe, President Franklin Delano Roosevelt—sixty-three years old and drained from a dozen years of stress in the White House—was sitting for his portrait at Warm Springs, Georgia. He suddenly said, "I have a terrific headache," and fell forward unconscious. Within a few hours he was dead of a massive cerebral hemorrhage, true apoplexy, and actually an uncommon form of stroke.

Vastly different was the experience of FDR's partner in World War II, Winston Churchill. In March 1953, at the age of seventy-nine, Churchill was going to meet with President Eisenhower in Bermuda when he was felled by a stroke. But by October the British Prime Minister had recovered and not long after was able to visit Washington. Although he retired from the prime-ministership in 1955, Churchill continued active in the House of Commons and even won another election in 1959. In the late 1950s he published his four-volume work, *A History of the English-Speaking Peoples,* and his death only came at the age of ninety-one, a dozen active years after his CVA.

Walt Whitman suffered a stroke with partial paralysis at the age of fifty-four, but that did not stop his creativity. In fact, he didn't put his *Leaves of Grass* into final form for another ten years. He also wrote the sixty-two poems of *November Boughs* and was heavily involved with many other activities until his death came—from a cause unrelated to his stroke—some twenty years later, in 1892. George Frederick Handel, too, was stricken by a CVA—at the age of fifty-two—yet continued to be immensely productive. Between the time of his stroke and his death twenty-one years later, in 1759, Handel produced some of his greatest operas and other works, including the magnificent oratorio *Messiah.*

Like these men, all of whom seem to have suffered from over-work and excessive stress, one of our greatest medical and scientific geniuses, Louis Pasteur, was also stricken by a CVA in the mid-stream of life. At the age of forty-six, Pasteur suffered a stroke so severe that he was comatose and was expected to die. As soon as he had regained consciousness, however, he insisted to those attending him: "I will not die. I have too much work unfinished!"

While still bedridden, Pasteur dictated a brilliant bacteriological technique. With his left leg paralyzed, left arm and fingers useless and bent, he returned to his laboratory, saying, "There is much work to be done." And he continued for nearly thirty years, until his death in 1895. During this time he was the first to prove that germs cause disease, created the basis for all modern aseptic surgery, founded the science of immunology and much more.

Stories of men like these are the best proof of how people can and do recover from stroke to lead a productive and worthwhile life.

The Hope in CVAs

While it is true that those we have just looked at were enormously creative people, the same thing can and has been accomplished by ordinary persons like you and me. And we have the advantage of skilled help today such as none of these men ever did. It is now clear that about three quarters of stroke deaths occur within the first ten days of the attack. To deal with CVAs, special care is available during this critical period. (We will discuss later what you should look for medically to ensure that any afflicted loved ones get such care and where you are likely to find it.)

But what are the chances of recovery today? Well, NINCDS experts say that among stroke survivors they have found that "30 percent have gone back to work or to their normal activity, with 55 percent disabled but capable of carrying on the activities of daily living, often with help. Fifteen percent are so helpless that total nursing care is required." However, new techniques such as bio-feedback promise an increase in those who can be restored to a functioning state, be able to use their limbs again. Experts estimate, too, that more than half of those stricken by CVAs have a degree of functional disability that is unnecessary in the light of the rehabilitation techniques available today. And it's now been proven that even after several years of lost function these limbs can often be restored to use once more.

FDR's stroke was too massive and severe to be helped. His doctors knew, of course, that his blood pressure had been dangerously high for some time, but back then, almost forty years ago, they lacked the expertise and the medications that physicians have at their command today—and which could probably have prevented this tragic and early death. Louis Pasteur might well have had his arm and leg restored to a usable degree today with the latest rehabilitative techniques—and the recurrence of his stroke would also likely have been preventable now.

Most exciting of all is the fact that today there are, for the first time, methods of actually *preventing* stroke. This is being done in a number of ways—by medication and by diet, by reducing the risk factors and even by highly sophisticated surgery. In short, the outlook for the knowledgeable person today is bright and much more positive than ever before.

But to understand all of this, we must begin by learning something about that place where strokes take place—the human brain.

2

THE BRAIN—
THE SOURCE OF STROKE

It is in the brain (the cerebrum) and its own blood vessels as well as those which bring blood to this organ that the source of stroke is to be found. Were this same damage to an organ's vascular (blood vessel) system to occur elsewhere in the body, the result would be vastly different: cut off blood supply to the heart and you have a heart attack, block the arteries to a small skin area and you might get an ulcer, and so on. But block those to the brain and you have massive damage to the body, destruction so varied and individual that—to paraphrase Gertrude Stein—a stroke is not a stroke is not a stroke; each one has its own peculiar character and symptoms.

The brain is man's claim to his uniqueness in the entire animal kingdom. Other animals run far more swiftly or have a keener sense of smell; eagles and hawks in full flight can see prey no larger than a rabbit dodging about in the brush a thousand feet below; seals can hear sounds at frequencies of 160,000 cycles per second (while even at birth man can only hear up to 30,000 and this drops rapidly until after the age of fifty he hears no more than 8,000). Only in the uniqueness of his cerebrum and central nervous system (brain and spinal cord) is man truly pre-eminent—and in his language and speech—so any damage to his brain serves to make him feel that much less of a human being while simultaneously depriving him of the full use of both mind and body.

But knowledge has been slow in coming, and only relatively recently, as man's history goes, has he learned where his mind and emotions are actually located. The Egyptians, who began embalming their dead five thousand years ago, treated and preserved the internal organs—heart, kidneys, intestine and the rest—with careful respect, but the brain was unceremoniously removed and discarded. This attitude toward the brain was common among the other ancients (Mesopotamians, Chinese, Hebrews and Hindus), who regarded the heart as the organ of man's intellect and emotions.

The Greeks of Aristotle's and Plato's time, however, were of two minds about this, some favoring the brain and others the heart as the site of the mind. Galen, Greek physician and founder of experimental physiology, first stressed the brain's importance, nearly two thousand years ago, but the ambivalent attitude lasted until Thomas Willis, great seventeenth-century British physician, studied the brain and nervous system and produced its most complete and accurate description up to that time. His discoveries of the blood circulation in the brain were to provide the basis for our understanding of how strokes occur.

Until modern times the brain remained a mysterious, little-understood organ to which a host of grotesque interpretations and theories were attached, often by the strangest people and for the oddest reasons. Amazing insights, intermingled with bizarre errors, have opened the way to our modern concepts. In the late eighteenth century an Austrian anatomist, Franz Joseph Gall, became convinced that mental functions were localized in special areas of the brain. He claimed that one could "read" an individual's intellect and personality by feeling the shape and bumps of the head, a practice he named "cranioscopy" and his followers called "phrenology."

Busts of the face, head and neck illustrating such areas on face and skull were still being advertised during World War I. Although Gall's phrenology died the death of all such fads, it did manage to arouse the interest of medical scientists in the brain. While it was shown that any bumps or irregularities on the skull has nothing to do with the brain tissue beneath, Gall's basic concept of specialized functions for certain brain areas was proved correct as early as 1861 by Paul Broca, a French surgeon who identified one of the speech centers (now known as "Broca's area") in the left half of the brain.

In fact, damage to Broca's area produces many of the speech and language difficulties that so often plague stroke victims.

Not long after Broca's work, Burt Green Wilder, professor of animal biology at Cornell University, started a brain collection to test the then popular theory that mental capacities—intelligence, talents and training—could be detected by examining the configurations of the surface of the cerebral cortex. A Cornell Brain Association was even formed to collect brain specimens of famous men and women in every field.

These Cornell scientists weighed and measured, checked the depths of the cortical convolutions and their lengths, all in search of some special developmental or anatomical differences in certain areas which would make it possible to distinguish a person's abilities or talents. The hope was to be able to tell a musician from a scientist, a painter from a poet. By the time Wilder retired in 1910 the collection comprised 430 brains, including those of "an erotic German" and of a murderer; of a physician, a poet, a thief and an alcoholic; of a famous psychologist, an economist and a pathologist.

One was even that of Helen Hamilton Gardener, prominent women's suffrage leader, born in 1853. Aroused by the statement of a New York neurologist and former U.S. Attorney General that a woman's brain was inferior to a man's, she embarked on an extensive study to disprove this and even wrote a book on it—*Sex in Brains*—which was translated into eight foreign languages. While Ms. Gardener's brain proved large and well developed, it was not as large as that of a compulsive murderer (believed to be the second largest on record).

In any case, Wilder's concept, like so many others before, simply faded away to disappear completely forty years ago and take its place as one of the many outmoded and disproven theories of the brain. However, not long ago Cornell resurrected from storage and put on display some two dozen of these preserved brains, for there has been a vast recent increase in scientific interest in this amazing human organ.

All these many if mistaken concepts of the brain did lead to serious scientific work, beginning with Broca. About the time of

Wilder's work, Santiago Ramón y Cajal, a Spanish histologist (one who studies microscopic anatomy), established the neuron, or nerve cell, as the basic unit of the brain and the nervous system. For this work Cajal gained the 1906 Nobel Prize for Physiology or Medicine. And with this breakthrough, neuroscientists began to dream of a complete solution of the mystery of the brain's functioning. But they looked to the answer as simply a matter of tracing out the nerve pathways like so many telephone wires—tedious and precise work, but readily realizable and only a matter of time.

This, too, has proved only the mistaken dream of an earlier and more naïve day when the knowledge of life processes, of medicine and science were on a much more simplistic, less sophisticated level. Today's electron microscope, for example, permits more than a million times' magnification, while ultrasensitive techniques reveal chemical reactions of a thousandth of a second in spaces of a millionth of an inch.

So it is that we now know that the study of the brain is a matter of learning about ultracomplex electrical and chemical phenomena taking place at incredible speeds in microscopic dimensions. In fact, a Stanford Medical School team recently searching for information about disorders in nerve cell function (as occurs, say, in epilepsy or stroke) have used microelectrodes with glass tips smaller than 1/25,000 inch. These can record electrical signals from within individual human nerve cells in bits of human brain which had to be removed from patients undergoing surgery for such cerebral disorders as epilepsy.

To fully understand the effects of a stroke one must appreciate precisely the elements of the brain, how these are put together and how they function; what the organ as a functional whole (the mind) is like and the difference between its sections; what the brain needs to survive and carry on its vital job properly—an incredibly complex task.

The Development of Your Amazing Brain

It all began 3.4 billion years ago, when the first known form of life appeared on this planet. Evidence that life is actually this old has only recently been uncovered in South Africa with the discovery of some two hundred cells so small they had to be enlarged 1,600 times just to be seen: four hundred of them stacked would come to no more than the thickness of a dime. Upper and lower fossil jaws found in the heart of Ethiopia by an international team of anthropologists headed by a professor from Cleveland's Case Western University seem to date the beginnings of man himself back to some five million years ago.

Neurons developed early in the evolution of animal life on this planet and they have not changed greatly in more than half a billion years. For it's about that long since the primitive neurons joined together to form the hydra's nervous system with its few hundred or thousand nerve cells. The first true brain appeared in the flatworm, perhaps more than 300,000 years ago. So it has taken a long time for man's magnificent brain to evolve, and its very complexity makes it vulnerable to the disruption produced by such disorders as stroke.

The Human Neuron

The individual neuron is the basic building block and functioning unit of your entire nervous system, including your brain. It is this cell which makes your whole body and mind work. These neurons are strange chubby cells with a wide variety of shapes and lengths (ranging up to several feet) but less than 1/100 inch in diameter. Almost unchanged for the last half billion years, the human neurons vary relatively little in nature and do not differ from those, say, of the lizard in either shape or function.

The cell body of the neuron is essentially a miniaturized chemical manufacturing system, one so active that it must be supplied with an estimated fifteen billion atoms of oxygen a second. Halt this oxygen supply for ten seconds, and the neuron is so affected that you lose consciousness; cut off its oxygen for five minutes or so, and this sensitive cell can be irreparably damaged or even die. This is why the loss of blood supply to any part of the brain in a stroke is so destructive to the human being and his brain—why even a reduction in the proper amount of oxygen and blood supply is enough to produce those passing stroke symptoms which mark the "little strokes."

The neuron is fundamentally a carrier of information, a transmitter of impulses. The sensory ones bring tales of sounds, sights, pain, body position and muscular movements so that your body can coordinate its complex multifaceted activities, its balance and its vital functions. The motor neurons carry commands to operate the muscles (for standing, walking, speaking, whatever), the glands and the other body structures. Most often there are a string of neurons which pass messages along to and from the brain and which, within that organ, spread information and prepare orders to go out.

Leading to each nerve-cell body are usually short filamentous extensions (dendrites) which bring messages into the neuron while there is generally a single long filament (the axon) coming out of the cell body. This axon carries the message (the neural impulse) on to the next neuron. But there is no actual physical contact between adjoining neurons, for the axon ends in a tiny knob that is separated from the dendrite of the next neuron by a gap of a millionth of an inch (a synapse).

A stimulus (a sound, touch, whatever) sets off the neural impulse (actually an electrical current), which then flows along dendrite, cell body and axon. When this reaches the end of the axon, the synaptic knob, it triggers the release of chemicals termed neurotransmitters. These flow across the synapse to open pores in the cell membrane of the dendrites of the next cell, trigger the impulse there and then set the message off again on the next step to its final target, somewhere deep in the brain.

Synapses are one-way switches which act as policemen to control the tens of thousands of impulses reaching the brain every second. A synapse can both fire and reset itself for the next impulse in about a thousandth of a second. Should this control break down, the flood of neural impulses can quickly overwhelm the brain and trigger an electrical storm across the cerebral surface, throwing the person into an epileptic seizure. And when these cerebral neurons and their synapses have been damaged in a stroke, just such epileptic seizures do occur.

The Human Brain

Your entire brain is only about the size of your fist—three pounds of deeply convoluted, indented and grooved shiny jelly. Yet the sheer enormity of what nature has condensed into this small package is truly startling. Your brain may contain as many as a hundred billion neurons, along with perhaps ten times as many glial cells, whose function is still not determined, although there is some indication that they may regulate neuronal nutrition.

A cubic inch of brain tissue contains a hundred million cells, a column the thickness of a pencil about fifty thousand neurons. And each of these neurons receives information from a thousand other nerve cells and passes this on to as many more. A typical neuron may have as many as ten thousand or more synapses and some may even have two hundred thousand. The total number of synapses in the brain remains imprecise but experts talk of between one hundred and five hundred trillion. So it is obvious how much disruption and sheer havoc can be wrought in so heavily populated an area by even the tiniest blood clot or destroyed patch of neurons.

To keep all these cells properly nourished, functioning and in good health requires a full fifth of the heart's output of blood as well as a fifth of the oxygen consumed by the entire body at rest. Cut off the supply of oxygen by cutting off the blood supply, and there may be damage to the deprived area—and unlike other tissues, any damage to the brain is irreparable and permanent. Once we have grown our full complement of neurons (by about the age of ten), that's it. We cannot replace damaged neurons or grow new ones—as, for example, we do with our skin, whose cells are often damaged or destroyed by cuts, burns or abrasions and then promptly replaced. Which is why the prevention of stroke is so very important.

Forming a wrinkled gray cover on your brain is your cerebral cortex (literally "bark" or "outer layer"), your "gray matter." It is only a tenth of an inch thick, and if stretched out, would be about three feet long and two feet wide. Yet in this small structure all conscious thought is produced; this is where your intelligence, reasoning, judgment, memory, will power and certain emotions reside. Here, too, is where voluntary muscle movements are controlled, where your senses are to be found (sight, hearing, taste, touch and smell), located in the motor and sensory areas of your cerebrum.

Your brain is made up of two halves, or hemispheres, with a vast network of connecting neurons to carry messages between. Generally, the two halves are symmetrical in their areas of sensory and motor specializations, with the right half of the brain dealing with the left side of the body, the left half of the brain with the right side of the body. However—and this is a vital distinction—they are not fully symmetrical in their functioning. Anatomical symmetry too can be seen, but this is not all that perfect and may be related to the specialized and different functioning of the two hemispheres.

The motor cortex, for example, is centered in a band of cortical tissue extending across the top of the brain from ear to ear with the sensory cortex parallel and just behind it. The cells here communicate with (either receive impulses and information from or send messages to) the body: adjacent areas of motor and sensory cortex respectively cover legs, knees, hands, face, and so on.

The left side of the brain has been considered the dominant one until very recently because most of us are right-handed and have Broca's and Wernicke's areas on the left side. (A decade after Broca's work Karl Wernicke, a German neurologist, located another speech center in the cerebral cortex of the left brain.)

Moreover, it's been shown recently that each hemisphere actually has its own and very special differences. The right hemisphere, for example, is the "dominant" one for music and for recognizing complex visual patterns.

This matter of right and left brains—"lateralization"—has stirred a great deal of interest in the last few years. The left brain is commonly regarded as the logical hemisphere, the reasoning one, which sees things analytically and in their separate elements. The right brain is the intuitive, the emotional and creative half, which sees things in their entirety and is concerned with total relationships. However, some experts now regard such sharp differentiation as being overly simplistic and see the relationship between the two brains as being the most important factor in our cerebral life.

But your brain is more than cortex alone. It is a sort of tiara, a tripartite unit of hindbrain, midbrain and forebrain which developed in roughly that order in the evolutionary process, starting in fact with the reptilian brain more than 300 hundred million years ago. The hindbrain takes care of such basic automatic and essential functions as keeping your heart beating and lungs breathing. The midbrain is small but important to your hearing and sight, and is believed to play a still somewhat unclear role in sleep and attention. The forebrain caps it all, both anatomically and evolutionally, for here is the cerebral cortex.

Yet even specific cortical centers are not that simple or discrete, for they all have connections and ramifications running through deeper layers of the brain, working with neuronal relay stations of higher and lower orders. It is the combination of many areas that results in the beautiful smooth cerebral functioning we normally display. A stroke can knock out virtually any spot however small in this system and so cause either minor or major disruptions. Take, for example, the thalamus at the base of the forebrain.

This is an integrating center, a telephone switchboard if you like, for all incoming information from the outside world and from within the body. Impulses from eye, ear, skin, gut, whatever, come into this thalamus to be joined, organized and passed on to the appropriate higher centers until, presumably, they reach the cortex, although neuronal pathways are almost inevitably lost to sight at some place or other in the vast confusion of neurons and synapses in the brain. However, should a CVA damage the thalamus, it can produce some of the most haunting and strangest pain sensations, as well as bizarre symptoms.

Or take the cerebellum, a large structure in the hindbrain. Often called the "secretary" of the brain, this structure coordinates muscle movement and balance, receiving information from the muscles themselves, the ears, eyes and tactile senses. Should a stroke affect this structure, the result will be abnormalities of movement and not abolition of movement (paralysis). By knowing the cerebral anatomy and functioning, the neurologist can pinpoint the site of the stroke from the symptoms the victim suffers.

The Importance of Speech

Speech and language go together like the proverbial horse and carriage. But it didn't begin all that long ago, for some say we only started talking fifty thousand years ago—that the power of speech is also the power to remember, to plan, even to think.

As Dr. Brudny puts it: "Thinking is actually silent speech, and without language we certainly wouldn't be what we are." Investigators today have monitored the electrical changes in the muscles of speech while subjects were thinking and have demonstrated we actually subvocalize (talk to ourselves without making sounds). In short, thinking is for many an organized form of silent speech.

With such deep significance to speech, it is easy to see how damaging its loss can be—and this inability to speak is a common occurrence in stroke. When the CVA affects the right side of the body it means the damage occurred on the left side of the brain—and this in turn is likely to affect the speech centers there. The exact location of the CVA—whether, for example, in Broca's or in Wernicke's area—will determine the kind and the extent of the speech problem (known as aphasia, something we will discuss in much greater detail later).

But now let us turn specifically to stroke, with this anatomy and role of the brain itself fixed in mind. In fact, the commonest cause of brain damage is stroke.

3

STROKES: THE KINDS, THE WARNING SIGNS AND THE SYMPTOMS

How They Occur and Their Frequency

A sixty-year-old New York professional man recently awoke one morning to find himself unable to use his right arm or leg, and when he tried to tell his wife he could utter only a string of garbled sounds. Following a heavy meal, a Midwestern woman executive in her late fifties complained of a severe headache and then collapsed, unconscious, her face beet-red and her breathing so heavy it was more like snoring. A retired East Coast blue-collar worker in his mid-sixties noticed a transient numbness and burning prickling sensations with some weakness in his left arm and leg. All these people had suffered strokes, of different types and degrees of seriousness. They would need different treatment but all required urgent and expert medical care.

NINCDS offers the best definition of this tragic disease: "A stroke is a sudden loss of brain function resulting from interference with the blood supply to the brain." Regardless of the actual disease process, the pathology involved, cutting off the blood supply to the brain for more than five minutes or so, invariably leads to some death of brain cells and impairment of function, to temporary or permanent loss of movement, thought, memory, speech or sensation.

Yet despite the seemingly sudden onset of this disorder, emphasized as it is by its very catastrophic and dramatic nature, the vast majority of strokes are actually only the end point of a nearly lifelong development of an underlying problem. The precursors of CVAs—the conditions known to lead to them—have been observed in our very young soldiers killed during recent wars, and may even be present in our children as well. However, the actual situation that produces such sudden damage to the brain can vary considerably. A stroke can be due to causes ranging from a weakened or burst artery to an occluded or blocked one, from one that is torn in an accident to one compressed by a blood clot or tumor.

The one thing that all strokes have in common is expressed in the scientifically preferred term for that disease, cerebrovascular accident, which describes both the pathology and the actual occurrence: in short, a condition in which something has abruptly and dynamically gone wrong with the cerebral vasculature (the blood vessel network of the brain), essentially either those arteries which supply blood to the head or those which carry it directly throughout the brain tissue itself. The phrases cerebral infarct, or infarction, are descriptive of the actual damage done to the brain tissue, the pathology involved. For an infarct or infarction is an area of dead tissue due to an interruption of its blood supply, although "infarction" is sometimes also used for the process.

The Blood Supply of the Brain

Blood is pumped to the brain through two pairs of arteries in the neck. The twin carotid arteries (right and left) run up the front of the neck, on either side of the windpipe, to enter the brain. Here each splits into an anterior (front) and middle cerebral artery, each of which then supplies its particular area of the brain. The two vertebral arteries (also right and left) are buried deep in the back of the neck, close to and on either side of the spinal column. When these vertebral arteries reach the brainstem (the base of the brain), they unite to form a single vessel called the basilar artery. This in turn splits to form the two posterior (back) cerebral arteries, one of which goes off to each side (to right and left) toward the back of the brain.

Each of these cerebral arteries is there to supply a certain area of brain tissue with blood, oxygen and nutrients (the brain uses 80 percent of all the sugar manufactured by the liver). Should one of these vessels be blocked by any of the stroke incidents, a specific area of the brain will be affected and a cerebral infarct result in the blood-starved section.

The neurologist has a detailed knowledge of the cerebral tasks carried out by each section (motor or sensory functions, speech or vision or balance or whatever) and the blood vessels which supply the areas. This specialist's physical examination of the patient will reveal any neurological deficits (loss or disability such as numbness, lack of muscle control, and so on): from this an expert knows which arteries have been affected.

Thus, if there should be an obstruction blocking the blood flow in one spot in the right anterior cerebral artery, the victim is likely to have muscular weakness on the left side—worst in the left leg, less so in the arm, and little if any in the face. On the other hand, if the blood flow in the right middle cerebral artery is seriously reduced, the weakness on the left side is likely to be most severe in the face and arm with little if any in the leg, but with some loss of vision. Should the left middle cerebral artery be affected, loss of speech may also occur. These impediments may also be accompanied by varied losses of sensation on the affected side as well. Blockage of the basilar artery is likely to produce effects on both sides of the body with such problems as facial paralysis, nausea, dizziness and loss of vision as well as various motor weaknesses and sensory losses.

Such bodily effects are due to cerebral infarcts—areas of dead neurons—resulting from the loss of blood supply. Specific effects also depend in part on whether large or small branches of the affected arteries are involved because this determines the size of the blood-starved area and so whether the resulting infarcts will be large or small. Then, too, the effects depend on whether specialized areas suffer infarction: should it be one of the speech centers, communication will be disrupted; should it be in the motor center for the right leg, this limb may be left partially or entirely useless. An infarct in the cerebral cortex will have one effect, one deep in the brain another, in the brainstem a third, and so on.

But nature has made an effort to protect your brain against vascular deficiencies by means of a cerebral arterial network called the circle of Willis, named for Dr. Thomas Willis. He described his circle in the mid-seventeenth century, and the original diagram of this structure was drawn for him by Sir Christopher Wren, whose masterpiece is St. Paul's Cathedral. Although one of England's most famous architects, he was also deeply involved in biology and medicine. In fact, he designed the first hypodermic syringe by attaching an animal bladder to a quill, and with this crude device gave intravenous injections to both dogs and humans.

This circle of Willis provides a vascular interchange at the brainstem to protect the brain should one of the four major supplying arteries coming up through the neck be blocked. The right and left carotid vessels connect with each other when they enter the brain by each sending out one small branch sideways to meet in the space between them. They also each send out a branch running backward to join two other small arteries (the right and left posterior cerebral arteries) which have come off the basilar artery and run to each side. The circle also has connections with the anterior and posterior cerebral vessels, so that blood flows upward from the circle through the cerebral arteries to the brain tissues as well as flowing around the circle itself.

Thus we have a continuous vascular pipeline at the base of the brain. This arterial circle connects the carotids to each other and to the basilar artery, which in turn is actually a continuation of the two vertebral arteries after they have entered the brain and joined together. In this way should any of these four main supplying neck arteries fail to bring in enough blood or become blocked, the brain may still be supplied adequately with its needed blood supply by way of the circle of Willis.

This is one of nature's fail-safe systems designed to provide backup mechanisms for its essential functions and tissues. Should a carotid or vertebral artery cease to bring in its full needed quota of blood, the vessels of the circle of Willis enlarge to carry more blood. This compensating increased blood flowing through the circle may supply sufficient blood to whichever cerebral vessels normally obtain their blood supply from the failing neck artery so that the affected brain tissue is not starved for blood.

While nature has done its best to ensure the brain's blood supply, this system is at best imperfect and often fails to prevent strokes, for three reasons. For one thing, little more than a quarter of strokes are due to a blockage of the major neck vessels. For another, the circle of Willis must be perfect, with its vessels in good condition, to take up what can be a very considerable slack. This isn't often so, because when some vessels such as the carotids are affected by hardening of the arteries or atherosclerosis, other vessels are likely to be affected the same way.

Finally, nearly half the population has so-called anomalies (defects or deviations from the normal) of the circle of Willis. The most common of these is the absence of a channel from the carotids to the basilar artery circulation, so that the two blood supply systems, anterior and posterior, cannot interchange as they normally do. The importance of this fail-safe system is evidenced in the fact that such anomalies are more common in stroke patients than in the population as a whole. Experts feel that these anomalies increase the chances of a stroke in persons with atherosclerosis.

The Ways Strokes Occur

There are a variety of incidents which can starve the brain by cutting off its blood supply and produce what we call strokes. These are the results of cerebrovascular diseases, and the chief kinds which produce strokes are considered the following:

1. By far the most common is thrombosis, or clot formation: a clot, or thrombus, forming in a cerebral artery, a carotid, vertebral or basilar artery can act like a plug in a hose, simply blocking the lumen (passageway) and preventing blood from getting through. The result will be a cerebral infarct in whatever area is supplied by the artery involved. If the vessel is a main one, the area affected will be large, but if a small one, it may be a matter of only a millimeter

(1/25 inch); such tiny ones are called lacunar infarcts. Autopsies commonly reveal small old cerebral infarcts in people who died of other causes unaware of the symptoms or effects of these small infarcts.

2. Closely related to this problem of thrombosis is that of embolism, or the obstruction of a blood vessel by any one of a variety of foreign bodies (a clump of bacteria, thrombus, air or whatever). In the brain this embolus, in the great majority of instances, is a blood clot which has broken loose from the wall of a blood vessel and been swept along in the bloodstream until it becomes wedged in the cerebral vessel where it blocks the flow. It is similar at this point in its effects to those produced by a thrombus.

3. Cerebral hemorrhages do their damage in a number of ways: the outpouring of blood into the surrounding brain tissue can destroy it by the actual local pressure; the break in the vessel can deprive the brain area it supplies simply because blood can't get through (as with a broken water hose); and the clot that forms can exert damage on surrounding brain tissue by pressure on it or on arteries, thus cutting off their blood flow.

4. Stenosis, or narrowing of an artery carrying blood to the brain, can obviously cut down the supply: this occlusion can be partial or complete, doing damage to the degree to which the vessel is blocked. Stenosis occurs when a tumor or blood clot presses on an artery and constricts it, reducing its lumen. Or stenosis can be due to atherosclerosis, whereby the passageway is steadily narrowed by the deposits formed on the inner arterial walls until eventually the artery can become totally occluded or stenosed.

5. Spasms were once considered a very significant problem but are not anymore. Today they are believed to do damage chiefly when there is cerebral hemorrhage and other vessels reflexly go into spasm.

The Figures on Strokes:
The Mortality and the Recurrences

Doctors generally divide the CVAs into two broad groups: the ischemic (lacking normal blood supply) cerebral infarctions and the intracranial (inside the skull) hemorrhages. These are considered separately because the two groups call for almost opposite medical and surgical care, are due to distinctly different processes and have markedly different prognoses.

Dr. Fletcher H. McDowell, professor of neurology at Cornell University Medical School, reports that of about a thousand CVA patients seen at the Cornell Division of New York's Bellevue Hospital, 88 percent had ischemic cerebral infarcts and only 12 percent intracranial hemorrhage. These figures coincide very closely with those of the Mayo Clinic group of epidemiologists who found the corresponding figures to be 85 and 15 percent. In seeking information about the relative frequency of cerebral thrombi and emboli among those suffering cerebral infarction, the Cornell group found that 92 percent suffered thromboses and only 8 percent emboli. The Mayo group again reported almost identical figures.

As to the recurrent episodes of stroke, the Mayo team found that 27 percent of stroke victims had recurrences, which again agrees closely with the Cornell figures. There is a wide variation in the mortality rates between those with ischemic cerebral infarcts and those with intracranial hemorrhages. The Mayo team found that 27 percent of those with infarcts died within thirty days of the attack, while the death rates of those with intracranial hemorrhages were roughly three times as high.

The Kinds of Strokes

A Los Angeles executive in his late fifties got into his car to drive to work one morning when he noticed that his right arm and hand felt numb and weak. Afraid to trust himself on those high-speed freeways, he called his doctor, who promptly rushed him to the hospital. Over the next several hours the symptoms steadily increased and spread until both the arm and leg on his right side were paralyzed while his speech became increasingly difficult to understand; it became clear both to him and to his wife that he had suffered a major stroke. In other cases a person may suddenly be paralyzed, or fall unconscious. And a Houston white-collar worker noticed that he had difficulty in saying words and felt marked tingling in his right arm, but it was all gone in a few minutes and he paid no more attention to it. Such different experiences represent the three kinds of strokes:

1. The Californian is typical of the "stroke-in-evolution," or progressing, stroke. In this kind, the paralysis and other impairments (sensory, communication and the rest) increase in number and severity gradually over a period of hours (one to five is characteristic) before the final and ultimate effects are reached. This may take up to two days to complete, and sometimes even a week, but this is rare.

The increase or onset of symptoms may appear in a series of steplike discrete ("stuttering") changes or in a pattern of unbroken continuum. Starting with mild weakness and numbness in a hand, one symptom after another or area of involvement may be added at a time, or the stroke may steadily spread from hand to arm and to leg until the whole side is paralyzed with sensations severely lost or altered along with other changes such as loss of speech and vision. The end result is a completed stroke.

2. The completed stroke is any CVA which has reached the point where there are no further sensory or motor losses. In cerebral embolism the full stroke comes on much more abruptly, and in cerebral hemorrhage it is likely to do the same. In cerebral thrombosis, however, the process is often slower, starting as a stroke-in-evolution. But regardless, the end point is the same. In a large number of patients with infarctions it was found that about a third of the victims had experienced a sudden onset of symptoms, and a fifth had symptoms that developed over a period of up to twelve hours. Only about one in twenty had strokes which took from twelve to twenty-four hours to reach completion. About a fifth of all those with infarctions had suffered the beginnings of their strokes during sleep.

3. The "little strokes" have become of increasing interest to physicians in the last decade, for they have proved to be warnings, in many cases, of what may later turn into completed strokes but can now often be prevented. Little strokes are generally distinguished from CVAs in terms of both time span and severity. Their symptoms are usually both more limited in nature and milder—as our Houston white-collar worker suffered—than cerebral infarctions, but the symptoms that appear may otherwise be similar.

Among the most significant diagnostic factors in little strokes is the time span involved. From the onset of symptoms until they reach their maximum, there is a lapse of less than five minutes and usually less than two; the symptoms commonly disappear in from two to thirty minutes, although they may last as long as twenty-four hours, but no more. Such conditions are termed *transient ischemic attacks,* or TIAs; they may be as mild as a drooping of the lip or a brief tingling in an arm or leg, and leave no disability in their wake.

However, strokes are also classified in another way:

1. A massive stroke is one in which there is a great deal of disruption of cerebral—and neurological—function. Arm, leg and facial paralysis may be virtually complete, there may be no sensation left on the affected side, and considerable vision may be lost as well. Should the CVA be on the left side of the brain, there may also be severe damage to communication—loss of ability to speak in any recognizable fashion, to understand what is being read or heard, loss perhaps of the capacity to add. Regardless of the side affected, vital cerebral functions (memory, for example) may be lost and there may be intellectual damage and even emotional problems. However, as we shall see in our chapter on rehabilitation, even victims of such massive strokes today may still regain a good deal of such extensive initial losses.

2. A light stroke is one in which there are only a few and not very severe neurological effects. These victims are the fortunate ones—and many CVAs are of this nature. These people can look forward to a recovery which will bring with it very little or no discernible disabilities.

The Warning Signs of a Stroke

Experts of the American Heart Association point out that your body itself may seek to warn you of an impending stroke and they urge you to learn this body language for your own protection. This is how these experts say your body may speak out to alert you of an impending serious CVA:

1. You may experience an abrupt transient weakness or numbness of face, arm or leg.

2. There may be some transient communication difficulties—a loss of speech perhaps, or some difficulty in speaking or in understanding the speech of others.

3. You may notice some difficulties with your sight—a sudden temporary loss of vision, say, or some dimness, particularly in one eye.

4. There may be an episode of double vision.

5. Unexplained headaches or a change in the usual headache patterns.

6. There may be a passing dizziness or unsteadiness.

7. You or your family may notice a sudden change in your personality or even your mental abilities.

In general the warning signals can include virtually any change in your neurological or cerebral functioning. This change would be reflected in such things as losing sensations (pain, touch), the use of body muscles (the ability to swallow, to make movements such as writing or facial expressions, even the ability to use hand or leg), and such very special human characteristics as the ability to communicate (to speak and read), to count perhaps or name the alphabet, to do a crossword puzzle, and so on.

How CVAs Strike, and What They Look Like

If the CVA should strike during sleep, its victim may be found unconscious in bed in the morning or may fall as he tries to get out of bed should one leg be paralyzed. If the stroke comes on during the waking hours, the victim may suddenly fall—either because he has become unconscious or because one leg suddenly turns so weak or is paralyzed so that it can no longer support him. NINCDS experts estimate that in about half the strokes there is some difficulty with speech—this and other problems of communication are generally termed *aphasia.*

The stroke victim may also suffer headache (probably the most common of all symptoms), dizziness, nausea, even a ringing in the ears, sometimes even before the actual stroke. He may lose consciousness for a short time, or may lapse directly into a coma, which may be due to a massive intracranial hemorrhage (as with FDR) or very extensive cerebral infarction (as evidently happened to Louis Pasteur). The longer a coma lasts, the poorer the outlook is for complete recovery from the CVA.

Most often, the face will droop on the affected side, the corner of the mouth sag and the eyelid not fully open. The affected arm and leg will hang limp, like that of a rag doll (what doctors term "flaccid paralysis"). Before long however this will change so that if the physician attempts to move a limb there will be a strong resistance (what doctors call "spasticity," or spastic paralysis): this creates a great deal of trouble and has proved very difficult to deal with in the past. This spasticity causes the affected arm to be bent at elbow and wrist, and the fingers curled. The leg on the paralyzed side may only be usable as a stiff supporting column. Should the victim try to walk, this leg has to be swung out wide to reach its next position. Once the foot comes off the ground it droops downward from the ankle, so that when you walk the toes drag on the ground.

Cerebral thrombosis, by far the most common form of stroke, is the most likely to occur during sleep and to develop gradually in a stuttering or steplike fashion. Cerebral emboli and hemorrhages particularly appear after some sudden strain or exertion (coughing, vomiting, a heavy meal). Usually there is no loss of consciousness at the onset of an ischemic infarction. Convulsive seizures at the onset are also rare, although they do occur in about 8 percent of stroke sufferers at some time during the acute and convalescent stages of the disorder. The most serious and damaging effect of stroke, many feel, is the aphasia and other communication problems that are so tragically common.

4

THE LOSS OF THE POWER OF SPEECH AND LANGUAGE (Aphasia and Dysarthria)

The Emotional and Psychological Effects of Stroke

When a stroke takes away the power of speech and language, those vital contacts with the surrounding world, there is invariably severe emotional and psychological trauma to both victim and family. The forms these take are many, complex and often seemingly bizarre—and truly seem to strike out of the blue. Today we often hear of people's loss of the use of their arms or legs and how they deal successfully with this—but few of us have any familiarity with those who lose the power of communication, are isolated in a world where they can't express thoughts, feelings, needs, wishes, or sometimes even understand what they themselves hear or read or see. Such an experience is made more terrifying by its very strangeness. It is thus only natural to include a discussion of the psychological problems as well.

The two primary speech disorders that result from stroke are aphasia and dysarthria (for more on the latter, see end of this chapter), but aphasia is by far the more frequent of the two. The CVA victim and his family and friends can only deal with this communications problem (what aphasia or dysarthria really is) by understanding the situation and how it comes about, whether it is likely to get worse, and what the future holds for such sufferers.

Appreciating the victim's and the the family's emotional reactions to both aphasia and to stroke helps the aphasic and the loved ones deal with these effects.

Aphasia

This word comes from the Greek and its literal meaning is "speechlessness." But to the stroke experts (the neurologists, rehabilitation specialists, speech pathologists and the rest) it means much more than just the loss of speech. Aphasia is a particularly tragic and terrifying aspect of stroke because it covers all four of our language components—speech, listening, reading and writing—as well as other vital areas of human communications such as gesturing. The aphasia victim may lose his capacity to count and spell, may no longer have the letters of the alphabet at his command, may not be able to tell time or recognize familiar objects or people, and much more.

Aphasia's devastating psychological impact comes not only from such losses but from the fact that it threatens the very biological core of the human being, his fifty-thousand-year-old power of speech. This has made him unique among the animals, given him his incomparable and remarkable flexibility as well as much of his intellect. Take speech away and you leave the human being isolated, unable to reach others; remove the other language components as well and he loses a vast deal of all contact with his fellow-men.

Imagine, if you will, suddenly awakening out of sleep to find that when you try to say something, a different word or phrase or a totally meaningless sentence comes out (for example, the aphasic person might say "cake" for "medicine," or "tomorrow blips the day whomever"). As Dr. Oscar Reinmuth, University of Pittsburgh stroke expert, recalls: "One of those fragmentary recollections I carry in my mind is of my Great-Uncle Bob, whom I saw only once when I was three or four years old. I was told he had had a stroke years before, and could not speak or raise his arm . . . I was misinformed—he *could* talk, but all he said was "Yes, yes, yes," over and over again."

The aphasic victim must endure and lose a great deal in his relations with the world. He is living in a whole new world where things said to him may sound like a totally foreign language which he has never even heard before—or he can't recognize his own wife or children. Confused, terrified, he easily becomes frustrated and intensely angry as he struggles to make himself understood or to understand what he himself says. He is likely to be markedly depressed and suffer a great deal of anxiety.

The effect of having one's world turned upside down this way can only barely be glimpsed by those who have never either personally had this devastating experience or seen others who have suffered through it. To gain a truly deep understanding and appreciation of what this experience entails, you should read a recent book called *Cry Babel* by April Oursler Armstrong.

April Armstrong is the daughter of the famous writer Fulton Oursler, with whom she co-authored *The Greatest Story Ever Told.* This courageous religious woman already had her doctorate in theology, was a well-known author and a college professor when, in 1972, she suffered a hemorrhagic stroke at the age of forty-six. She awoke from surgery to find that when she struggled to speak, all that came out was a babel of nonsense, and with vulgarities. As she herself says in her introduction: "All my language skills— speech, writing, understanding, and reading were gone . . . There were only seven real words left in my brain."

This detailed record of her experiences and struggle to successfully recover will surely be immensely valuable to other aphasics and their families. She recalls that she didn't know what "husband" meant, had lost her knowledge of the alphabet, her ability to spell, do crossword puzzles, for example, and arithmetic. Written during her recovery, this brilliant woman tells what aphasia can do—and how it can be defeated with time, effort and belief. But how modern medicine successfully helps and treats this condition will be left for our detailed chapter on recovery and rehabilitation.

What makes it all so horrible is that the typical aphasic is perfectly normal mentally and fully aware that he or she has lost (temporarily at least) so much of the capacity to communicate and live a normal intellectual life. He is aware of what he wants to say, but is shocked to hear something quite different issuing from his mouth. He may curse, use vile language, spout senseless jargon or the words may be perfectly correct but strung together in such a way that what is said ends up being meaningless. The aphasic may not even understand what he himself is saying. Or there may be a whole host of other distortions, losses and damages to our intricate and complex language abilities and means of communication.

Finally, these losses—in speech, say, or reading, or writing, or understanding—may be of different degrees. There may be much more loss of speech and understanding than, say, of writing—or some of these may be lost and others left undamaged. Aphasia, like so much else of stroke, is a highly individualized affair, since it is due to the variable damage done to the brain by the widely different infarctions or hemorrhages that occur.

The Anatomy of Aphasia

Our knowledge of the anatomical basis of aphasia actually goes back to 1861 when the great French neurologist Paul Broca described his fifty-one-year-old patient who was able to understand perfectly anything that was being said to him, yet his speech was such that he could not be understood. In a post-mortem examination Broca found destruction of a part of this man's left cerebral cortex, which lies roughly in front of the ear. The French neurologist then amazed his contemporaries by showing them that this was limited to the left side—for if this same area on the right side of the brain were damaged there was no aphasia.

Broca's area is adjacent to that part of the cerebral cortex which controls the muscles of the face, jaw, tongue and throat. Because of this proximity, any infarction or hemorrhage which damages Broca's area will almost always produce a marked paralysis of the right-hand side of the face, jaw, mouth and throat as well. This has helped to prove that aphasia is not due to any loss of muscular control: this same muscular paralysis is produced on the left side of the face if a right brain infarct occurs in the area corresponding to that of Broca's area on the left side—but there is no aphasia. Moreover, the muscles of speech can obviously continue to operate normally in Broca's aphasia, for these same victims can still sing, often beautifully, and certainly their problems with grammar cannot be due to muscular problems.

The victim of Broca's aphasia speaks in a very slow, labored fashion and cannot put together adequately formed grammatical sentences. As Ms. Nina M. Hill, assistant director of the Speech and Hearing Institute of New York's ICD Rehabilitation and Research Center, a speech pathologist and aphasia expert, explains about these patients: "In describing how to make scrambled eggs, he will say slowly and with great effort—'egg . . . crack 'em . . . uh, uh, uh . . . white thing . . . uh . . . break it . . . uh . . . spoon . . . stove . . . uh, uh . . . eat . . .' These aphasics are only able to retrieve with ease the content words of the language—can only use the nouns and verbs but not the grammatical words that make for the normal flow of speech."

Damage to Wernicke's area, however, produces a wholly different kind of aphasia—one in which words may be spoken in sentences that are well put together and are spoken with ease but actually mean nothing. The speech of a Wernicke's aphasic is not unlike the double talk that once was used by some comedians with nonsense syllable or words buried in their fluently spoken sentences.

Damage to Wernicke's area can also result in so-called word deafness (doctors call this "auditory receptive aphasia"). In this condition it's as if you heard a word in a foreign language you don't understand or one tapped out in Morse code—the sounds are plainly heard but they have no meaning.

On the other hand, disruption of the neural fibers connecting Broca's and Wernicke's areas can itself lead to disturbances of speech even if the two areas remain intact and unharmed. However, where speech has been affected, writing is invariably disrupted too—but precisely what cerebral centers or neural tracts are involved in writing still remain unknown. In fact, infarctions or hemorrhages that injure Wernicke's area can disorganize the use of language entirely, affecting speech, writing and reading.

An amazing and only poorly understood ability we all have is really intriguing to brain experts who still don't understand how we can recognize people even though they may change substantially in appearance over the years, or how we can pick out a small familiar face with a quick glance at a picture of a large mass of people. There are a pair of narrow bands of cortical tissue on the undersurface of the two hemispheres whose task it apparently is to accomplish this very recognition. We feel this is so because if that tissue is damaged by a stroke, the victim will not recognize his own spouse or child or oldest friend—yet he will be able to immediately identify the person by listening to his voice.

For a long time there has been a belief in hemispheric dominance —that there is a superiority of one cerebral hemisphere (one brain, if you will) over the other. This has essentially been based on the seeming fact that one brain has more specialized functions—and those of speech and language in particular—than the other. The left brain has, accordingly, been regarded as the dominant one because its speech and language centers were thought to be unilateral (one-sided) only.

In the animal kingdom only man is known to have this hemispheric dominance. Such cerebral dominance seemed to be further proved by the fact that well over 95 percent of aphasias are due to left brain damage (strokes in particular, but also to injuries and surgery). Furthermore, about 93 percent of human beings are right-handed—and of these at least 99 percent have their speech and language centers (Broca's and Wernicke's areas) in their left cerebral hemisphere.

New discoveries in the neurosciences are beginning to challenge such flat statements, and perhaps the future will even see marked changes in this thinking. Some of this recent thinking may well offer considerable new hope and promise for those stroke victims who suffer aphasia. In fact, experts have increasingly noted that with modern methods, considerable recovery of language abilities is possible even in those whose CVAs seriously damaged their speech centers.

As we've seen, neurons cannot regenerate once they are destroyed by infarction or hemorrhages. But there is now increasing evidence that the functions of the destroyed areas can be taken over by other neural tissues either adjoining or perhaps even in the opposite brain. These alternate areas may well simply always be there—a passive backup, as it were, available for use should the original primary specialized areas in the dominant hemisphere be damaged. For example, it has recently been demonstrated that some specialized areas have fringe tissues which can take up the burden should the original areas be damaged and no longer be able to carry out their tasks. There is new evidence too that this may even be true of Broca's aphasia—that if the infarction or hemorrhage here is not too large, the chances of recovery of speech are quite good.

This hemispheric dominance is not entirely clear in those who are left-handed or ambidextrous. Such people can be made aphasic by damage in either hemisphere, although the disabilities are more lasting when the left brain is involved. Moreover, those who have had such left-brain damage in early childhood usually end up with their speech centers in their right brain.

It has also been noted that certain aphasic patients do better than others: children, especially those under eight years of age, often recover remarkably well; left-handers are more likely to recover than right-handers (and even among these, those with left-handed parents, sisters, brothers or even children have a better chance than those without left-handed relatives). All of which would seem to indicate that there is some relation between which hand you use and which side of your brain is the dominant one. So your handedness may well influence your chances of recovery from an aphasia should you suffer a stroke and be saddled with this problem.

Doubts about the absolute dominance of one brain over the other have just been substantiated in Dallas and Boston. At both University of Texas Southwestern and Harvard Medical School, neurologists report evidence that the right brain also has certain dominant language functions all its own. The right hemisphere would seem to contribute the pitch, rhythm and stress in pronunciation and voice that add the quality of emotion to one's speech, for damage to the right brain left the patients studied without the ability to make the tone of their voices convey their mood (anger, annoyance, determination, sorrow, happiness) to listeners, as our voices normally do.

One of the patients observed was a teacher in her thirties who had suffered a stroke affecting her right brain. Although she was able to go back to her teaching a month or so afterward, she found herself with not one but two communication disabilities. For one thing, her voice was weak and did not project adequately, but the more damaging encumbrance was an inability to express emotion: her facial expressions and her gestures lacked force and animation, and her voice failed to convey the emotional quality that normal speech carries.

So marked was this that she found she could no longer maintain classroom discipline because her speech failed to express her feelings of anger, determination or other emotional qualities. In fact, even her own children weren't sure when she really "meant business." Even adding a "Damn it—I mean it" didn't help because the expletive too came out in an unemotional, flat monotone.

This stroke victim found she had even lost the capacity to cry or laugh. When she tried to cry it sounded unconvincing and stilted; and when she forced a smile or laugh it appeared artificial. All this even though inwardly she felt sad or happy, as the case might be. It was six months before the ability to express emotion, to put coloring and volume into her voice began to return. And eventually it took eight months before she could use her voice once more to get across her feelings; before she could express her emotions with facial expressions and gestures, could laugh and cry normally once more.

Dr. Elliott Ross, professor of neurology at the University of Texas and one of those who reported these cases, sums up their importance: "This is the first time a disorder of emotional language production has been correlated to a focal [localized] lesion [wound or injury]." From these cases, Ross has helped to introduce the concept that the right brain becomes the dominant one in contributing the emotional component to communication, and as he puts it: "One could view the division of language functions between the two hemispheres of the brain as the left being responsible for what you say and the right being responsible for how you say it."

The Outlook for Those with Aphasia

As we have seen, aphasia and its language difficulties have nothing to do with mental or intellectual qualities and do not affect the mind. This very fact helps to make the condition doubly traumatic to the sufferer, for since he is almost invariably aware of the problem, it makes him even more disturbed.

Next, of course, is the fear that aphasia will continue to worsen. But this does not happen, simply because once the stroke is complete, it has, along with the other effects, almost always reached its worst point. However, when the victim is overly tired or tense or depressed, the aphasia may become more marked. But then, all our language talents (speech and the rest) are likely to suffer even in perfectly normal people in times of stress, exhaustion or depression.

One of the first questions asked, too, is whether aphasia may be a passing thing, might disappear by itself. The answer here is a strong "Yes!"—for over half of those who suffer aphasia recover completely during the first days or weeks following their CVA— they have what doctors call "transient aphasia." In fact, both President Eisenhower and Prime Minister Churchill had transient aphasia. Eisenhower even recovered so quickly that he was able, shortly after his stroke, to joke about the difficulties he had found with certain words, and there was practically no trace of his aphasia later when it had passed. The nation was greatly relieved to hear this, for his stroke occurred at the very beginning of his second term in the White House and actually, when he died twelve years later, it was of a heart attack and not a stroke.

Getting over aphasia is a very individual matter, but most experts feel that the greatest degree of recovery occurs during the first year. It may and often does continue at a much slower pace thereafter, with many achieving success only after several years. Some observers have suggested that speech recovery takes place by itself within a three-month period, but that thereafter only formal therapy will help.

The Kinds of Aphasia

As we have seen in discussing the anatomy of this problem, many areas of the brain (and, it would seem likely, both brains as well) are involved. The more areas or regions that are essential to any normal cerebral function, the more open the mechanism is to disruption—and communication involves a wide variety of places many of which have not yet been traced or identified. So a stroke hitting any one of them can disturb speech, language or communication, which is likely why aphasia is such a frequent complication or effect of stroke. Also, some of these language areas deal with a wide range of closely interrelated but still different facets of the complex, highly developed human system of communication. Which means that, as we have already seen, a stroke can produce many different kinds and forms of aphasia, depending on the site of the damage. And although patients with aphasia usually demonstrate some impairment of all four language components (speech, hearing, reading and writing), the degree of disability may vary considerably among these in any one person (speech poor, hearing fine, and so on). In severe aphasia, for example, all recognition of words, pictures or objects may be lost, while other components may vary.

Both the knowledge and the concepts of aphasia are growing and changing rapidly, and so is the classification of these disorders. Much of current thinking regards the aphasic's problem as a loss of memory. And this faculty, memory, must itself be divided into retention or storage of what has been learned, and recall or retrieval of information (bringing it into the conscious mind, where you can use it). The aphasic's problem may lie in one of both of these areas: he may lose part of what he has stored or he may lose the ability to retrieve certain things. Thus, in Broca's aphasia we saw the inability to retrieve for use those grammatical expressions that connect our words in speech and permit a normal and fully adequate sentence structure.

As Ms. Hill describes it: "During the first six months or year after the stroke there is more of a blockage than a loss. Ask the patient what a cup of coffee is and he can't say it in words. But if

I sing 'Let's have another cup of . . .' he will say 'coffee.' The word is not lost forever, but it's a question of how the patient can best retrieve it."

She explains about anomia, the classical form of aphasia: "Anomia is a word-retrieval problem for content words, nouns and verbs, and is very common to all aphasics. It's like a word on the tip of your tongue—it's right there and you'd recognize it if you heard it, but the aphasic may only be able to retrieve the initial letter or the number of syllables, or some idea about the word, knowing that that's not it. Just imagine every time you open your mouth there will be at least two words in every sentence that you'll have anomia for—that's the frustration of aphasia."

Then, too, there are the so-called paraphasias, or phonemic paraphasias, another aspect of this same problem. These are what we would in normal persons consider an unintentional transposition of sounds called spoonerisms (after Oxford's William Spooner, who was famous for such slips of the tongue as "half-warmed fish" for "half-formed wish"). In these problems the aphasic will substitute one sound for another. This can be so severe that the victim may call a table a hubstool or substitute one word for another—soap for sink, boy for girl, even yes for no.

Experts classify the aphasias in two ways. They can be separated into expressive or motor aphasia and the receptive or sensory kind. Broca's aphasia is typical of the expressive and Wernicke's of the sensory kind. When the problem is an expressive-receptive aphasia it is sometimes termed a global aphasia and is caused by the destruction of a large part of the left brain. In this global form the victim can say only a few words at the most, can understand only a few simple words or phrases, can neither read nor write.

Experts may also classify aphasias as fluent or non-fluent depending on the flow of the victim's speech, the use of uninterrupted phrases and sentences. A non-fluent aphasic has a slow speech with pauses and hesitations, often with incomplete sentences. Broca's aphasia is one example of the non-fluent kind. On the other hand, the fluent aphasics have a normal rate of speech and use full sentences but often have fewer nouns they can retrieve, use incorrect or reversed syllables in their words and may even have a completely unintelligble speech. Fluent aphasics also generally have difficulties in understanding speech.

There are other facets of aphasia as well. For one thing, victims who speak more than one language find their native one much easier to use. Aphasics may still be able to count or recite the alphabet or the days of the week—forms of automatic speech similar to our "Hello" or "How are you"—even though they are severely aphasic otherwise.

Writing is often disturbed and the aphasic makes the same errors in writing that he does in speaking. Thus, misspellings, omissions and an inability to form the individual letters are common. Personal difficulties vary widely, for some can only write their name while others can only copy words but not write spontaneously. Some can write the letters of words adequately but not be able to put them down in correct order. Still others cannot write legibly at all. In those with less impairment, spontaneous writing may be reasonably accurate but slow and sparse.

Dysarthria

Dysarthria is another form of disordered speech—but this condition is due to damage to the motor or muscular control of speech. Here the cerebral damage has taken place in a different area of the brain from the aphasics. Dysarthria damages speech by affecting the muscles involved, just as the stroke causes paralysis of an arm or a leg—in short, the effect is due to the muscles rather than the way aphasia interferes with the mind itself. Speech may be slow and slurred with low pitch and a harshness of the voice, or the speed, loudness and rhythm may be altered. Strokes producing this may involve brain areas quite apart from the speech centers or even the cerebral cortex.

The Emotional and Psychological Effects of Stroke

Dr. James C. Folsom, director of ICD Rehabilitation and Research Center, warns that "the first impact of stroke on the family and on the individual comes when he recovers consciousness or when he realizes he has had a stroke—and it's devastating. I think the basic problem of stroke is the effect it has on the family—everything else, no matter what, ends up being the residual of this. This is why I feel so strongly that these people need to get involved with some crisis intervention, some family education."

The first step toward resolution of the devastating emotional impact of a stroke lies in understanding how and why it has such psychological impact. However, there is help available and in the better stroke facilities—in stroke units and centers, in advanced rehabilitation centers—provision is made for the psychological help needed by patient and family alike. Psychologists and psychiatrists are there to evaluate the emotional impact and to deal with these reactions. Such help should be actively sought by families when they are not suggested by the medical personnel, or form part of the treatment. Crisis intervention is a new mental health approach designed to help survivors of catastrophes such as floods, earthquakes, major fires. And strokes certainly belong in this very same category—for patient and family members alike.

Family relationships—between husband and wife, parent and child, individual and family as a whole—are like a seesaw. When the individual on one side changes, becomes stronger or weaker, ceases to act as housekeeper or breadwinner or whatever, the seesaw balance shifts and tilts. Those on each side must seek a different and more secure perch as the weight at either end changes. Both parties become uncertain and shaky as they strive to find a new relative position, to establish a new balance, as they feel threatened for fear of falling off, of the relationship abruptly ending.

Help is needed to reorganize this balance, to re-establish new relationships and new family patterns. The breadwinning role may have to pass from one set of hands to another, care of the house may be altered, a healthy active person may now find himself in a dependent role with activities of the family markedly changed.

All of us have certain unconscious pictures of our own bodies, what psychiatrists term "body image." This is formed early on from the things we learn about ourselves—and from the attitudes of the society in which we live, the importance placed on appearance, health, activity and age. In fact, the American attitude toward aging—its depiction of the older person as weak and useless, as a "crock" or "crone" or "over the hill"—leaves Americans terrified of aging and desperately trying to avoid and deny its presence.

Dr. Robert N. Butler, director of our National Institute on Aging, explains: "Americans suffer from a personal and institutionalized prejudice against older people. Although this may be a primitive universal dread of aging, true in all cultures, it is reinforced and thus more striking in our own."

Thus when the stroke victim must see—at least at first—a devastating physical disability, paralysis of as much as half his body with a loss of sensation as well, he is terrified. Add to this—so often—an aphasia, and you have a terrifying feeling of helplessness, of isolation. There are feelings, commonly, of one's body and strength breaking down, and a frightening shift in body image. It's enough to make the young victim feel old, particularly since stroke is traditionally thought of as an old man's disease. This is particularly insidious since most stroke victims are in their sixties and beyond, emphasizing the societal attitude—and so necessarily their own—toward the aged, and resulting in feelings of self-anger, loss of self-esteem and depression.

Many victims view their attack as the first step on a short road to death; there is a need to cope with this new body image which must now often include paralysis, loss of sensations, aphasia and sometimes even sexual impotence (a common by-product of the inevitable depression that results from such catastrophes); there is bewilderment, frustration, anxiety and self-anger or rage as well as guilt feelings. It all can result in panic and disorganized behavior. Fear of death and insanity may become major preoccupations of the stroke victim.

The underlying problem and the reactions of patient and family are to a very large extent dependent on their personality structures, the ways in which they deal with life in general, and separation and loss in particular. Separation is surely the most basic and painful of all human experiences; it starts with the trauma of birth—the first, the prototype of separations—leaving the protective warmth and stability of the womb. That first wailing cry is a protest against the pain of separation and loss—and all future separations and losses will stir up these feelings and the pain.

In stroke one loses much: the ability to move and to feel parts of one's body, perhaps the capacity to speak, understand speech, see. The older persons—those in their sixties and beyond—have already suffered the losses of age (like youth, physical strength) which are of themselves difficult to deal with. And now they have the losses of a stroke to deal with as well. For the young and the middle-aged there is the implication of aging inherent in this disorder as well as the loss of all the activities they may value so much.

Dr. Pietro Castelnuovo-Tedesco, professor of psychiatry at Vanderbilt University, explains in connection with all this: "You are faced with the issue of loss throughout life and it has to be dealt with over and over again. This leaves both sadness and a great deal of resentment associated with the loss. All of us would like to feel we are somehow capable of stemming the tide of aging, accidents, and all sorts of dire events which can overtake us—and finally, the death of the organism which represents the full obliteration of the self." All of which explains the devastating emotional impact of stroke.

Having such knowledge makes for self-understanding and thus the ability to cope with the natural psychological reactions. This also helps the family to understand how to reassure the victim himself. "The biggest problem about stroke is the expectation that nothing can be done," Dr. Folsom warns us. As we shall see later, this is not true. A great deal can be done today—another form of reassurance to be given the stroke patient. Dr. Folsom also urges that family and professionals all work together to reduce the confusion and disorientation of these sufferers by simply stating the hopeful facts whenever the occasion arises—that the victim's condition is good, that he is being taken care of and will be protected, that the outlook is hopeful.

The Psychological Reactions of the Stroke Victims

Anxiety is common following CVAs, often shown by the victim's increased emotional tension and feelings of impending doom. Anger, too, is present and often directed at someone in the family or the hospital staff. Any frustration provokes anger in human beings (why we wrench at a door or drawer that sticks), and there certainly is a great deal of it in stroke. By understanding this it is possible to view the patient's anger with equanimity, without taking it personally or responding in anger.

Depression, too, is almost universally present and arises out of the self-anger and lowered self-esteem felt by the stroke victims. They may deny depression but will admit they can't control their own behavior. This depression may well be behind the fact that nearly all stroke victims cry easily and often seemingly without reason. While all this is no cause for special concern and will usually disappear, psychiatric or psychological aid can be of enormous help to both patient and family to smooth the way.

Stroke victims usually lose their temper as never before, even push or slap others in their frustration and anger. They may also "act like a child," but most of us tend to do that when we are ill, for any disability tends to make human beings regress to a greater or lesser degree. The family can aggravate or help this situation, and expert advice is needed here too.

The family of a stroke victim is likely to be troubled by a host of perfectly normal but difficult-to-deal-with emotional problems of their own. There is anger at the sick person (a normal reaction to the vast difficulties such illnesses present) and guilt feelings because of this anger and perhaps also because unconsciously the family sees it as their fault. The worries, new responsibilities, changing familial relationships and other troubles all help to produce tensions, stresses, anxieties and depression in the family.

Dr. Folsom urges help—in the form of crisis intervention—for family and patient alike. Crises of this sort can do serious and lasting emotional damage to human beings. Every way of preventing this should be sought out. The professionals who are available in stroke units or rehabilitation teams and how they can help are dealt with in detail in our chapter on rehabilitation. But should a stroke situation prove excessively stressful and emotionally traumatic, the family and patient might do well to consider seeking regular psychiatric help to bring it under control because such problems may not only delay and prevent recovery but also precipitate physical illnesses in all concerned.

5

THE LITTLE STROKES
AND THE STROKES OF
CHILDREN

These two aspects of stroke may seem modern discoveries to medical profession and lay public alike, but actually both have long been known. Almost two thousand years ago Soranus of Ephesus—the founder of obstetrics and gynecology, biographer of Hippocrates—noticed that even though "apoplexy" usually struck without warning, dizziness and a ringing in the ears would ofttimes foreshadow an attack, could even be regarded as its precursor. In the eighteenth and nineteenth centuries a few shrewd medical observers, too, became aware of such warning signs. One of these physicians even recognized that episodes of transient paralysis which appeared and repeated themselves were in some way the harbingers of a later "apoplectic" attack.

In the Louvre there is a painting of a young boy by the early-seventeenth-century Spanish artist Jusepe de Ribera. This youngster's right hand is pictured in the contracted and curled position that is so typical of stroke; also, his mouth droops and he carries a sign explaining that he cannot speak. Evidently the artist recognized the patterns of childhood stroke long before the medical profession did. It is often forgotten, too, that famous Sigmund Freud, in 1897, wrote a classical monograph on infantile hemiplegia in which he described these strokes in detail. He even noted that it struck those "from a few months of age to three years of age."

Both the little strokes (transient ischemic attacks) and childhood strokes are important: TIAs because they can act as a forewarning of the risk of future strokes which today can be prevented; childhood strokes because they must be recognized if the child is not to grow up into a scarred and seriously damaged adult.

The Little Strokes (the TIAs)

In his mid-fifties, a harried New York businessman noticed he had difficulty speaking clearly, a tingling numbness in his right arm. It was all gone within five minutes, and although it did reappear two or three times, he ignored it, assuming it was overwork and tension. And a Midwestern woman in her early sixties was troubled with occasional spells of blindness (like a curtain descending over her right eye) which came on very quickly and lasted no more than a minute or so. The woman sought medical care, but the man did not —until he suffered a stroke and aphasia. Yet there are measures available that doctors can and do take to actually prevent those with TIAs (which is what these two suffered) from going on to the tragedy of completed strokes.

It is only in the last three decades that the medical profession has become aware of and deeply concerned over such transient ischemic attacks. Only in this period have doctors begun to fully realize the meaning of these episodes, to recognize the threat of a completed stroke which they carry, and to learn how these TIAs present an opportunity for physicians to step in for the first time, and actually prevent completed strokes.

Until 1950, doctors believed that cerebrovascular spasms were the cause of TIAs. But about that time the role of atherosclerosis of the four major neck arteries in contributing to cerebral infarctions was first recognized. Atherosclerotic plaques and clots, it was also realized, could form and enlarge on the arterial walls until they closed down the blood channels of these major neck vessels, and so interfered with the blood supply to the brain that they caused TIAs.

About this same time, too, the role of microemboli (microscopic emboli) in causing TIAs was also suggested—that such tiny bits of material broke off from the atherosclerotic plaques in these neck arteries. These emboli then float along through the cerebral blood vessels until they lodge temporarily in some artery to stop the blood flow sufficiently to produce the symptoms of TIAs. The process that produces atherosclerosis and its plaques, the clots and emboli, is a complex affair.

Yet even today, as Dr. J. P. Mohr, University of South Alabama professor of neurology and stroke expert, explains: "A major underlying problem is the continuing uncertainty of the mechanisms of TIAs. If there are several mechanisms, the risk for stroke and the therapy might well differ for each type, a finding that could resolve much of the conflicting data on the subject."

A TIA, being an episode of cerebral dysfunction, of temporary neurological deficits, can produce, in miniature—a little stroke—any of the symptoms of completed strokes. But the two deciding factors in the definition and diagnosis of a TIA are that it will have completely disappeared within twenty-four hours, and that it leaves no persistent or permanent neurological deficit.

In a very real sense, and more than with a major stroke, the TIAs are invariably "bolts from the blue" in many ways. The onset of the symptoms is startlingly rapid, going from no symptoms at all to their full variety and intensity in less than five minutes, and usually in less than one. The duration of such attacks varies. As we have seen, it usually lasts only two to fifteen or perhaps thirty minutes, although on occasion it may persist for as long as twenty-four hours. The resolution or disappearance of each episode of attack is correspondingly swift, ordinarily taking a few minutes at most and leaving no residue, no symptoms or changes, to mark its appearance or passage.

The frequency also varies—there may be only a single episode or multiple attacks at different intervals. The most dramatic of the TIAs are the kind suffered by the Midwestern woman mentioned above. Her sudden monocular blindness is termed by doctors "amaurosis fugax": the onset of its symptoms is a matter of ten to fifteen seconds and its resolution and return to normal is just as swift. This visual condition is one of the situations that has provided proof that microemboli are the cause of TIAs because doctors have been able to see clumps of blood platelets or other emboli actually moving through the retinal blood vessels.

The eye provides doctors with the only clear window by which they can see the body's vascular system in actual operation without having to cut into the body to expose such vessels. By looking through the transparent lens of your eye with a microscope (as your ophthalmologist often does in his examinations), the physician can clearly see the blood vessels of the retina. In the Midwestern woman's amaurosis fugax the doctors observed these clumps actually blocking the blood flow momentarily as they slowly worked their way through the retinal blood vessels.

The Kinds and the Importance of the Little Strokes

The TIAs, classified by their source, are divided into two groups: those due to problems in the carotid arterial system (which supplies the anterior and middle cerebral arteries), and those related to the vertebral-basilar arterial system (the vertebrals fuse to form the basilar artery and supply the posterior cerebral arteries). Any emboli set loose in carotids or vertebrals will reach the cerebral areas supplied by the particular neck vessel involved, so that experts can tell from the TIA symptoms where the underlying vascular problem lies, whether it is due to microemboli or atherosclerotic changes in these vessels or stenosis from these same changes.

This differentiation between these vascular systems is important for two reasons. For one thing, there is a distinct difference in the prognosis of the TIAs originating in these two systems. And, for another, the treatment of the problems of these two systems is also quite different. There can even be differences when there are physical reasons for their TIAs.

It is simple for surgeons to expose and operate on the carotids in the neck. But it is virtually impossible to do any surgery on the vertebrals because of their deeply buried position adjoining the spine, and the fact that they often pass through bony rings as well. As a result of their anatomical locations there can be differing mechanical problems. Trauma (an injury)—a blow on the neck, a belt or harness that suddenly tightens—can cut off the blood flow through the carotids, which are covered only by soft tissue of the neck. But the vertebrals can be affected by arthritic bony spurs on the spine squeezing these vessels to reduce their blood flow, even cutting it off should the individual move his neck or bend his head in some special way. In fact, even under ordinary circumstances the vertebral arteries can be kinked and blocked with sharp head or neck bends.

Most important of all, naturally, is the significance of these TIAs. Of themselves they would seem minor, since episodes do pass quickly without leaving any residue. But it is their close involvement with subsequent strokes that make TIAs so important. However, as Dr. Mohr points out: "The frustrating nonuniformity in definitions and methods used to collect and analyze data on TIAs has defeated the most exhaustive attempts to bring order out of seeming chaos in our literature."

Only some figures are clear. TIAs seem to strike people during what many consider their most productive years of life. A number of studies agree that nearly half of all TIA victims are between the ages of fifty-six and sixty-five, and roughly a quarter between forty-six and fifty-five, with the preponderance of the rest being among the elderly. Twice as many men as women are affected. And one study of a biracial community in Georgia found twice as high an incidence of TIAs among whites as among blacks, and this preponderance of whites has been confirmed by others. It has been suggested that this may be due to the fact that atherosclerosis of the neck arteries is less common among blacks.

The reported incidence of completed stroke in a series of patients who had suffered TIAs has varied from 12 to 62 percent. It's been estimated that three years after their first attack, one third of untreated TIA sufferers will already have suffered a stroke, one third will still be having TIA episodes, and one third will no longer be having them. A Mayo Clinic study has found that almost exactly one third of those with TIAs went on to completed strokes during a three-to-eight year follow-up, with the risk of stroke being highest in the first year, about 23 percent. It's also been estimated that the chances of those with TIAs having strokes after the first year is sixteen times that of those who have never had a TIA. It's also been estimated that from 25 to 50 percent of those who have a TIA will have more than that single attack.

What worries these sufferers is, naturally, the prospect of untimely death. Another Mayo Clinic study of a series of TIA patients followed over a period of some fifteen years has revealed that the mortality rate rose steadily over this period to reach a startling 60 percent, but some observers feel that simple aging may account in part for this terribly high rate. Other studies, with shorter follow-up periods, have found mortality rates ranging roughly from 15 to 25 percent. The problems that have lead to such sharply different figures are at least in part due to the confusion over diagnoses.

But let us now look at the picture and the figures from another angle. Two of America's leading stroke experts—Dr. Clark H. Millikan, professor of neurology at the University of Utah, and Cornell's Dr. Fletcher H. McDowell—agree in saying that "transient ischemic attacks are the most important warning symptoms of impending stroke. They occur in up to one half of all patients who develop stroke." And another Mayo Clinic study has recently shown that nearly twice as many victims had carotid TIAs as had vertebral-basilar ones: the survival rates for these two groups were the same and there was no significant difference in the likelihood that they would go on to completed strokes.

Others have also found that about three quarters of those who suffered completed strokes in the carotid–middle-cerebral area had previous TIAs affecting this same territory, indicating the importance of considering TIAs from the point of view of their source. Obviously some of these are more sinister than others and warrant more radical intervention and more concern.

The Symptoms of TIAs

It is important to know both the seriousness and the consequences of strokes—to protect your life. Drs. Millikan and McDowell warn that among those who suffer TIAs, less than half actually seek medical help before they suffer their strokes (as did our New York businessman). So to protect yourself it is necessary both to be familiar with the symptoms of TIAs and to realize that if you experience such an episode, you should promptly seek medical help.

The diagnosis of a little stroke depends primarily on the physician's interpretation of his patient's recitation of what happened, for most TIAs are long gone when the doctor sees the patient. It is important to be aware that specialized help may be needed. Recently a special team made an extensive study of nearly fifteen hundred patients who either were suspected of suffering from TIAs following an examination and history taking by a physician in the emergency room or outpatient clinic in six medical institutions, had been hospitalized with a diagnosis of TIA or had been referred to a neurologist for diagnosis of suspected TIA. The initial diagnosis of TIA by a non-neurologist was confirmed in 39 percent, ruled out in 30 percent and left unestablished in another 30 percent.

These institutions had been carefully chosen to provide a national picture of good medical care and included such places as Boston's Massachusetts General Hospital, Seattle's University of Washington, Indianapolis' Indiana University School of Medicine. The final diagnoses by neurologists were then checked in three ways and confirmed in 84 to 93 percent. The most common mistake in diagnosis proved to be completed strokes in which neurological deficits had been missed until specialized neurological examinations were conducted.

The team concludes that its study pointed up the need for greater knowledge by the general medical profession about TIAs. It would seem to indicate that those with TIAs might do well to ask for a neurological consultation if their general practicioner diagnoses a little stroke. As this team also points out—mistaken diagnoses of TIAs may result in unnecessary and sometimes dangerous tests, unneeded diagnostic studies, and even dangerous forms of treatment, as well as introducing the possibility that the recognition and treatment of other and life-threatening medical problems may be unduly delayed.

The symptoms of TIAs can best be classified as has the NINCDS Study Group on TIAs—with the clear understanding that these occur as we have described in their time, onset, duration and disappearance, and occur (as do all strokes) on the side opposite the affected cerebral hemisphere. The symptoms of the TIAs of the *carotid arterial system* this Study Group, and others, find are:

1. Motor disturbance: May be weakness, paralysis or clumsiness (a "heaviness") of arm or leg or face (or all) on one side.

2. Sensory defects: Numbness, loss of sensation or so-called paresthesias (altered sensations such as tingling, pins-and-needles, burning) in limbs or face (or both) on one side.

3. Aphasia: Any of those problems we mentioned already.

4. Loss of vision in one eye or a part of one eye.

5. Homonymous hemianopia: Loss of one half of the corresponding visual field in both eyes (upper or lower half, right or left).

6. Any combination of these: When the motor or sensory disturbances occur they do so all at once unlike the steplike, or stuttering, appearance so common in strokes-in-evolution.

The symptoms of the *vertebral-basilar artery system* differ sharply because they involve the areas covered by the vertebral and basilar arteries, which are sometimes bilateral (both-sided):

1. Motor disturbance: This may be weakness, paralysis or clumsiness in one or more limbs in differing combinations and degrees in all four limbs up to quadriplegia, sometimes shifting from side to side with different attacks and varying from slight losses to paralysis. Even the facial muscles on one or both sides may be affected.

2. Sensory defects: Numbness, loss of sensations and paresthesias in any combination of the limbs up to all four, and usually involving one or both sides of face, mouth or tongue; sometimes changing from side to side with different strokes.

3. Visual loss: Complete or partial loss in the corresponding halves of both retinas.

4. Homonymous hemianopia: similar to that of carotid system.

5. Double vision, inability to arrange words in an understandable way, dysarthria or dizziness (with or without nausea and vomiting).

Where TIAs are set off by some exercise or particular body movements, the physician has a clue to the cause and can even have the opportunity to see the TIA on command, as it were. Changes of head or body position, or arm exercises, which precipitate a TIA are almost invariably due to their creation of a mechanical obstruction—a kinking or bony pressure—of the vertebral artery. But the ultimate diagnosis of TIAs are not always easy, and as we have seen, may call for the expertise of the specialist, the neurologist. Many of the techniques used in diagnosis of completed strokes may be needed (the problems and techniques are so entwined and complex that they are best left for our later chapters).

The Treatment of Little Strokes

This is a combination of medical and surgical approaches, often no different from those used for completed strokes, but the successful treatment of TIAs can and does prevent such strokes. One of the most exciting advances is very new—the use of a simple household remedy which can actually cut the incidence of completed strokes from TIAs in half, in men at least. This truly miraculous drug is none other than plain old aspirin.

But the complicated background reasons for the use and selection of either drugs or surgery must be explored first so that these therapeutic measures can be understood and readers be able to evaluate the choices should they be faced with them. And many of the drugs require careful choices and precise laboratory procedures to monitor their use. The surgery itself is complex, performed with microscopes in a variety of different procedures.

The Strokes of Children

"A previously healthy child . . . suddenly becomes ill. . . . The initial symptoms may be violent, with fever convulsions, or vomiting . . . speech impediment and aphasia are frequent . . . sooner or later . . . epileptic seizures occur." So wrote Sigmund Freud in 1897 when he described infantile hemiplegia, strokes in children, in his classical monograph. Yet the concept of strokes in children and infants, even those in the womb, is so startling even to professionals that it may cause errors, as the NINCDS Strokes in Children Study Group warns: "The belief that stroke threatens only those in the twilight of life when blood vessels have lost vitality and are obstructed with atheromatous deposits is widespread. Even more incredible to many is the possibility that a neonate [newborn infant] can be the victim of a stroke. . . . Too often the neurologically impaired child is given the nebulous label of brain damage or cerebral palsy."

True, strokes in children are much less common than in adults but when they do occur they can be as devastating, with considerable weakness or paralysis and often complicated by convulsive seizures, and may even be fatal. On the other hand, Dr. Gerald S. Golden, professor of pediatrics at the University of Texas, says that only rarely does aphasia persist in children. And in our chapter on aphasia we have seen how the speech center will shift to the uninjured right side in children afflicted by this disorder.

The past twenty years have seen vast strides in medicine with the development of a whole flock of subspecialties revolving around children—pediatric neurology and neurosurgery, rehabilitation for children, and the like. It is vital for parents to be aware of this so that, should they be so unfortunate as to have their child involved in this tragedy, they can seek help not even available from the usual specialist in these problems.

It has now been widely recognized that, medically, children are a far cry from being small adults and one age group even differs from another, with the hemiplegic infant presenting a wholly different set of medical and rehabilitative problems than, say, the six-year-old. The fetus, the neonate and the child are all at different developmental stages of their nervous systems and brains, which are far more plastic and adaptable than, say, the adult's—and this offers much more hope but demands more attention.

Most children with stroke do not die directly from the disorder itself. But they are left with a variety of neurological and brain damage that can be terribly crippling to the child's chances of living a normal, satisfying life. The problems will be physical, psychological, social, educational, and eventually those of adjustment to the world where he will have to make a living and survive. The child can indeed suffer all the deficits we have already mentioned in connection with adult strokes: paralysis, weakness, visual loss, aphasia, crippled self-image. So special is this problem that we must look at it in more detail.

The Causes of Childhood Stroke

The NINCDS Study Group feels that the majority of strokes in children are more likely to have unknown causes than known identifiable ones. For example, hypertension (high blood pressure) in children has only recently come in for serious consideration, and along with it has come the awareness that children too are subject to atherosclerosis. Although both these conditions are major factors in adult strokes, there is no conclusive proof as yet that they lead to strokes in children.

Leukemia and hemophilia can both lead to hemorrhagic strokes. Either local or systemic (generalized) infections can also cause infantile hemiplegia: this can occur as a direct effect (meningitis and other local infections can lead to thrombosis in cerebral arteries) or as a complication of bacterial heart infections (endocarditis). Mayo Clinic investigators have shown that this endocarditis leads to hemorrhagic strokes, and other researchers have shown that it causes cerebral infarction.

Trauma (injury) is another source, for this can cut off the blood supply through the carotids, by producing a carotid thrombosis or clot. Aneurysms (ballooned weak spots in an artery's wall) can rupture and set off severe brain hemorrhages, although these are rather rare. Even a very few instances of migraine with its constricted arteries have been reported as resulting in infantile hemiplegia. Sickle-cell anemia is another disease considered to be a cause of childhood stroke, but some experts find that this usually occurs in older children and adolescents.

Infantile hemiplegia is, as with the adult kind, commonly due to thrombosis or embolism, but injuries to head and neck are one of the most frequent causes of these. The thrombotic occlusions can arise from a variety of causes in children, but not always very clear ones. In the cerebral vessels these causes have included calcification in the arterial walls, and infections (brain abscesses and meningitis, for example). Occlusion of the carotid in a child is most often due to trauma, such as an external blow (even compressing the artery against the spine) or a pointed instrument penetrating to the vessel, but sometimes it occurs with no evident cause. There has frequently been some local or systemic infection (pharyngitis, for example).

Emboli causing strokes in children are usually the result of some heart or lung condition, and most commonly affect the carotid and middle cerebral arteries. Rheumatic heart conditions or actual cardiac bacterial infections are causes, as are lung infections. Brain hemorrhages in children are commonly due to malformations of the cerebral vascular system or to aneurysms.

The Symptoms, the Outlook and the Treatments

In arterial thrombosis, a previously well child, usually under two years of age, suddenly suffers weakness or paralysis of the arm or leg or face on one side with all the symptoms of the adult stroke including aphasia. However, it may begin with seizures or be accompanied by severe convulsions and even coma. Occasionally, too, it may begin with a series of transient episodes which finally culminate in a completed stroke. Cerebral embolism begins with characteristic suddenness and may be similar in its symptoms. Experts emphasize that stroke in infants and children produces a very wide range both in the symptoms themselves and in their degree (from a slight passing weakness of muscles to severe spastic paralysis).

Strokes in children are fortunately rare, but they can be serious and may leave a variety of aftereffects, so that parents are naturally concerned about the prognosis of any such tragedy. If the CVA strikes the left brain, it can produce aphasia, but in those under four years of age this usually disappears, although there may be some residual deficits or difficulties (in the articulation of speech, for example). In children between four and eight years of age there may be some mild language disability persisting, but after this age permanent difficulties are common.

Epilepsy, with recurrent seizures or convulsions, affects roughly half of these children. The attacks usually appear within the first year after the stroke, although they may start much later. The younger the child at the time of the stroke, the greater the risk there is of such seizures. But if none has developed by the time the child is eleven years old, it is considered very unlikely that he will have a convulsion. In fact, less than 20 percent of those children who had their stroke begin without convulsions ever develop epilepsy. The convulsions in the beginning may likely be due to the immaturity of the child's nervous system which often does respond to any difficulty with convulsions—as parents of children who have had a high fever from even minor illnesses can testify.

Roughly half of these hemiplegic children do have some motor deficiencies, and the younger the child afflicted with a stroke, the greater the likelihood that an affected arm or leg will be underdeveloped. In cerebral embolism the outlook is not nearly as bright as with thrombosis because it usually occurs as a result of heart disease and can have a 25 percent mortality rate, with half its survivors suffering severe neurological deficiencies. In intracranial hemorrhages, too, the ultimate result depends on the underlying problem. With ruptured aneurysms there has been a 50 percent mortality rate. But there is hope that increasing medical and surgical expertise will improve this picture in the years to come.

One thing that concerns doctors and parents alike is the effect of stroke on the intellect and personality of these young developing human beings. The NINCDS Study Group says that these children's physical problems are usually such that normal schooling is possible but that their intellectual, perceptual (vision, hearing—their aphasias, in short) and behavioral shortcomings are such that special schooling may be needed.

Among the children who have suffered strokes there are a few with superior intelligence, but most have some mild intellectual deficiencies, and roughly a quarter or so are actually retarded. Perceptual difficulties—especially visual ones—often create additional learning and psychological problems. Finally, there are the behavioral problems such children are left with and these are manifested in a variety of ways such as hyperactivity, limited attention span, poor ability to tolerate frustration, ready outbursts of rage, impulsivity, and the like.

Psychological Help and Rehabilitation

These two aspects go together, for the hemiplegic child should have one with the other. The child's body is much more plastic and adaptable than the adult's—which makes for both good and potentially bad results. Compared with the adult, the child can look forward to better development of compensatory neural pathways in the damaged brain. On the other hand, any neuromuscular deficiencies—muscular imbalance or weakness, say—can produce considerable more skeletal deformity than in the adult. Rehabilitation thus assumes a very vital role in preventing deformities and in helping the child to learn, or relearn, the use of his own body. The techniques involved are not markedly different from those used with adults, so we will discuss all of them together in our chapter on rehabilitation.

Fortunately, today there is much more awareness of the problems of the disabled and there is greater sensitivity toward the deficient child—and toward his parents in their suffering as well. Great as the fear is which the adult experiences in his stroke, it is much worse for the child, who hasn't the background of maturity and life to support him in this experience; he is suddenly faced with an inability to use his body or to experience things as he is accustomed to, and is abruptly removed from home and parents to the very strange and frightening hospital environment.

The child may regard this as a punishment for something he's done wrong, adding guilt to all the other psychological problems faced at this time. He may even feel he will never return to family and home again. All this can have a vast effect on his personality in many ways and at many levels.

Parents, too, suffer at this time—as well as do any brothers or sisters. They may feel guilt and anger, and serious problems arise as parents have to face the possibility of permanent physical and mental disabilities. This is even more traumatic when they finally learn that there is no cure or hope. It is important to remember that there is considerable understanding available among the experts in the field of rehabilitation medicine and the social sciences. Emotional help is vital for family and child alike if they are to recover from this traumatic experience. Help is needed to re-establish a family relationship in which the parents can find comfort and pleasure, and the child grow to the maximum its new deficits will allow.

Psychological counseling is invaluable at this time and psychiatric help may be needed, depending in considerable part on the emotional background and problems of all involved. The specialized medical facilities which care for these hemiplegic children are likely to have group sessions for parents—another reason why such specialized care should be sought. These group sessions can prove very helpful and supportive to the newly involved family, which can discover that their problems are no different than those of others who have suffered this before, that their feelings are common to all who find themselves in such tragic circumstances, and perhaps most important of all, that they are not alone. Often many practical suggestions come out of such sessions to make dealing with the common problem easier and more successful.

II

PROTECTING YOURSELF FROM STROKE

6

THE CAUSES OF STROKES AND HOW TO PROTECT YOURSELF (PART I):

Atherosclerosis; the Risk Factors and How to Reduce Them

Oral Contraceptives, Diet, Cigarettes, etc.

Atherosclerosis (often referred to as "hardening of the arteries") is the most common of the serious chronic diseases afflicting people both in America and in the other technologically advanced nations. Its complications *can* be fatal—they are actually the leading cause of death in the United States—but if not, they are the chief reason for visits to physicians, days spent in the hospital, and limitations of physical activity. In 1975 (long before our wild inflation) this disease was costing the economy more than $50 billion a year in lost productivity and wages and for the expenses of medical care.

The two chief complications of atherosclerosis are heart attack and stroke. These two cardiovascular diseases alone kill more Americans each year than all our other causes of death put together. In fact, experts at our National Heart, Lung, and Blood Institute (NHLBI) say that atherosclerosis "is directly involved in 87 percent of deaths from cardiovascular disease."

Actually atherosclerosis is a complex disease whose precise nature and all of whose aspects have not yet been either fully explored or entirely understood. However, there is general agreement that atherosclerosis is the most common underlying problem in stroke, although the exact mechanism involved in each instance may vary. In the Cornell-Bellevue study of nearly a thousand stroke patients, 92 percent of those with ischemic cerebral infarction (due to thrombi and emboli) had cerebral atherosclerosis. Thrombus formation, however, may involve more than just atherosclerosis, and blood-clot formation may be that additional element.

We can only hope that an understanding of the causes of stroke will show us the way to prevent it—and many experts feel we have already reached the point at which we can successfully take preventive measures. This is why we are devoting both this and the next chapter to a detailed exploration of the causes of stroke. Here we will look at both the disease, atherosclerosis, the way it develops and the risk factors of stroke. Even more important, we will examine the way some experts believe atherosclerosis can be prevented and perhaps even reversed after it has developed.

The problem of atherosclerosis is a complex one that involves all of us. One Mayo study alone indicates the degree to which we are all affected. Of a hundred autopsies selected at random, the Mayo team found that forty of these people has suffered atherosclerotic stenosis to an extent of 50 percent or more in at least one major neck artery. In other words, the brain in almost half these individuals had been receiving only half or less of the normal blood supply through one or more carotid or vertebral artery.

Every one of these autopsied people revealed some degree of atherosclerosis in at least one of their neck arteries. Since only sixteen of these forty with severe stenosis of their neck arteries had marked cerebral infarcts, it would indicate how many of us may be functioning marginally, perhaps just getting by without CVAs until some other problem causes death. But it wouldn't take much to tip such a fragile balance. Moreover, even three of the sixty with seemingly minimal atherosclosis did suffer such strokes, so it would seem we would all do well to avoid atherosclerosis as much as possible.

As Dr. McDowell points out, stroke victims do have the most severe atherosclerosis, but there are also severe cerebral infarcts in those with moderate or perhaps only little atherosclerosis. On the other hand, those with extensive atherosclerosis do sometimes manage to get by without strokes. But the tie-in between atherosclerosis and stroke is clearly there and in a number of ways.

Susceptibility to stroke also arises out of what are known as "risk factors" from which you can learn ways to protect yourself. Certain characteristics of human beings, their life styles and environments are known to increase the danger of developing particular diseases—these are what doctors call risk factors. Implicit in this concept is the belief that the presence, magnitude and duration of one of these factors (diet, environment, inherited traits) in an individual increase the likelihood of his falling prey to the particular disorder.

As important or even more important, this belief also implies the other side of the coin—namely, that eliminating or reducing certain risk factors may make it possible to prevent the disease, a concept we shall explore so that you may be able to avoid these risk factors and thus protect yourself from the tragedy of stroke.

The Story of Atherosclerosis

Actually, atherosclerosis is a disease of one's whole lifetime. It is a disorder that starts very early in life, in infancy in fact, and slowly and insidiously progresses. All too often, by the time the disease is recognized, its victim is dead from a stroke or a heart attack. So it is not surprising that atherosclerosis has emerged as the number-one killer in most industrialized countries. Prime examples, along with the United States, are Canada, England, Sweden, Australia and West Germany.

We know it is an ancient disease, for it is present in the Egyptian mummies of the twenty-first dynasty, some three thousand years ago. It was not much later that the Greeks discovered that the pulsation of the arteries was due to their muscular coats. And the Chinese have long checked the pulse strength and rate as a test of health and disease. One can well assume that with the many shrewd medical observers down through the centuries, some of them must have noticed the difference in feel when the arteries hardened with atherosclerosis.

This disease, in the form of its complications, has long been studied, and the sixteenth- and seventeenth-century anatomists provided a good deal of information. But it was not until two hundred years ago that Antonio Scarpa, professor of anatomy in Pavia, recognized that changes took place in the inner lining (the "intima") of the arteries in this disease.

Atherosclerosis is now known to affect the intima of large and medium-sized arteries, turning what should be a thin, flexible muscular blood-vessel wall into a thickened, rigid one. It gives no sign of its presence but begins with an obscure abnormality of the arterial wall in very early life. Typically it remains silent and symptomless for a long time—until it affects a vital artery, shutting down its blood flow and creating a major bodily disaster such as a stroke or heart attack. As the experts at NHLBI put it: "The precipitating factors that convert the insidious process in the vessel wall from morbid [diseased] anatomy to a clinical catastrophe are not entirely clear."

What is known, however, is that the basic lesion (the circumscribed pathological change) is the so-called atheroma or atheromatous plaque. These plaques look like pearly-gray mounds of tissue which change the smooth intimal surface into a roughened raised and uneven wall. These plaques can vary in diameter from several millimeters (one is 1/25 inch) to a centimeter (4/10 inch). They protrude into the lumen, or blood channel, of the artery where they can interfere with the flow of blood. Should these plaques grow to a point where they occlude the lumen and totally block the blood supply, they can produce either a heart attack or a stroke.

These atheromatous plaques usually consist of a core of lipid (cholesterol and other fats) covered by a cap of fibrous or scar tissue. The mechanism by which this fundamental lesion first forms and then grows is still unclear. However, many of the medical scientists interested in atherosclerosis feel that these plaques begin as yellowish fatty streaks in the walls of arteries.

These fatty streaks are first seen in the aorta, the body's main artery, which comes directly out of the heart, and through which all blood is funneled before it passes through ever smaller arteries on its path to the distant organs and tissues which it must supply. Actually, these fatty streaks are present in the aortas of nearly every child by the time he reaches the age of three. The coronary arteries are the ones that supply the heart muscle, and fatty streaks usually make their appearance in these vital vessels between the ages of ten and fifteen, and grow in size up to about the age of twenty-five. They usually do not appear in the cerebral arteries until about the age of thirty-five.

These fatty streaks produce no symptoms of themselves and their only known meaning or importance lies in the concern that they are either the precursors of the plaques or will develop into them. Confusing the picture, however, such streaks have been found in the arteries of all peoples that have been studied for this formation—regardless of what the incidence or prevalence of atherosclerosis is in the older years among these particular peoples. Moreover, except for the coronary arteries, the extent or degree of these fatty streaks has no correlation with the degree of atherosclerosis which may appear at some later time in life.

Animal experiments have taught scientists a lot about the process of atherosclerosis. For example, nearly twenty years ago a Southern scientist discovered that a New Orleans Zoo baboon which was being routinely autopsied turned out to have atherosclerosis, and the species has been used ever since to study this disease experimentally. Fatty streaks, for example, can be produced in many animals fed on a diet high in fat and cholesterol to raise the level of the blood lipids (a group of fats easily stored and used as sources of fuel in the body) to produce the condition termed hyperlipidemia (an excess of fats or lipids in the blood). The fatty streaks in humans and animals appear similar, and the lipid found present in them is cholesterol.

This ability to create fatty streaks in animals by creating an artifially induced hyperlipidemia provides experimental proof that elevated blood lipids tend to increase their deposition in the arterial walls. Even though some of these streaks do not develop into plaques, the fact is that some precede the plaques and will be found in the same anatomic sites as atheromas—in the coronary arteries, for example. This has led many medical scientists working with these problems to conclude that these streaks really are the precursors of atheromatous plaques.

The widespread nature of atherosclerosis has been proved by repeated studies of autopsy results showing that 80 to 90 percent of all adults have a significant amount of atherosclerosis. The decade of the seventies brought new understandings and new concepts about the way these atheromatous lesions develop and progress. As a result, NHLBI experts feel that there are four fundamental biological phenomena which make up the chief components in the development and progression of these atheromatous lesions in the affected arteries:

1.   An increase and proliferation in the numbers of the smooth muscle cells in the intima
2.   Synthesis and formation of fibrous connective tissue by the smooth muscle cells
3.   The passage of lipoproteins (a complex of lipid and protein molecules in the blood) into the intima
4.   The metabolism (all chemical changes occurring to substances inside the body) of lipids and lipoproteins and their relationships to the smooth muscle cells in the arterial walls

One of the puzzling parts of atherosclerosis is the way some lesions regress and heal, while others simply continue spreading and developing by the further increase of smooth muscle cells and the deposition of lipids and connective tissue in the arterial walls. There must clearly be some factors present which determine the path this process will follow, whether to healing and regression or to growth and progression.

But the most fundamental part of the process—what the actual initiating factors of mechanisms are—still puzzles investigators. The most common hypothesis is that some injury to the inner lining of the arterial wall triggers a sequence of events of considerable complexity which changes the whole arterial picture. This "injury" could be something so minor that all it really does is change the permeability of the cells lining the arterial lumen (the so-called endothelium). Such an altered permeability could allow substances normally controlled to enter the walls and produce a deposition of fatty substances like cholesterol.

Another situation might be a severe injury in which the lining or endothelial cells are detached at some weak point where the force of the blood is especially powerful, as in an arterial bifurcation. The exposed underlying tissues would then attract special blood cells called platelets, which are involved with the formation of blood clots.

His research into this problem leads Dr. Russell Ross, professor of pathology at the University of Washington, to see the process thus: "Our hypothesis would suggest that if the 'injury' is a single event, then the lesions can regress, and thus would be silent in terms of clinical sequelae. On the other hand, if, as we believe to be the case, the 'injury' occurs chronically or is repeated many many times over a period of years, the lesions would become slowly progressive until they reach the point of sufficiently occluding the lumen of the artery so that thrombosis occurs. If the artery is an important one in maintaining the vascular supply of a critical organ such as the heart or the brain, then myocardial infarcts (heart attacks) or cerebral infarcts (strokes) would occur."

Dr. Ross has shown experimentally how atherosclerosis might arise in humans and might explain the advantages of certain protective dietary measures widely advocated today. He deliberately injured the endothelial cells in a primate, using a catheter introduced into the selected artery. The animal was simultaneously fed a high-cholesterol diet, so that its blood cholesterol was in the same range as that of human beings with hypercholesterolemia (hyperlipidemia, with cholesterol the fat involved). Lesions that then appeared were identical with those which are the classical precursors of human atherosclerosis. However, if the blood levels of cholesterol are not high and the injury is not repeated, the lesions will regress and disappear. But if the blood cholesterol levels are high and the injury repeated, the lesions will become progressive.

Returning to man: What if an injury occurs to the endothelial lining of a human artery? We have already outlined the anatomical changes that may take place in four steps outlined by NHLBI experts and believed to lead directly to lesion development. Following this pattern, we might anticipate a loss of the endothelial barriers, an increased permeability, smooth muscle-cell proliferation, connective-tissue formation, entry of lipids, and blood-platelet adherence to the defect in the wall. The result of all this will be a protrusion of tissue into the lumen of the vessel from its endothelial lining—the atheromatous plaque.

Like human fingerprints, no two of these plaques are identical. Such atherosclerotic plaques are composed of fibrin (an elastic protein making up the essential portion of a blood clot) and other elements of connective tissue, endothelial cells, varying amounts of lipid (especially cholesterol), dead cells, and perhaps platelets, and possibly calcium deposits as well. On this rough surface, platelets will accumulate and form further thrombi, or clots.

Sudden total occlusion of the vessel can occur should platelets stick to the surface to form a thrombus which becomes so large as to fill the lumen. This blockage can also come about as the result of a rupture of the plaque with its materials spewing out into the lumen to disturb the blood flow. Disturbed and slowed blood flow is likely to cause platelets to collect and stick to each other to form a clot. Finally, too, the arterial wall may now be so weakened by plaque formation destroying the healthy elasticity that the wall bursts under arterial blood pressure (particularly if this should be abnormally high, as in hypertension) and a hemorrhagic stroke results.

Finally, too, emboli may form as bits of thrombi break off before they have become fibrous and formed a hard, firm plaque. This can even block the lumen or become emboli to be swept along in the blood current. Such emboli may then lodge somewhere in a tiny artery or one whose lumen has also been so narrowed by plaque that the embolus is too large to be carried through by the bloodstream. This then becomes an embolic stroke, an ischemic cerebral infarction.

Lipids, cholesterol and their relatives have been mentioned here and there, so the time has come to discuss these. But first a note about a study to which we will be referring more and more. In order to gain much-needed scientific epidemiologic and clinical information on heart disease and stroke, the Framingham Study was begun over thirty years ago.

A group of over five thousand men and women between the ages of thirty and sixty-two, free of cardiovascular disease, were selected in the town of Framingham, Massachusetts. Each of these volunteers reported every two years for medical examinations, but neither diet, life style nor other environmental factors were altered, although information on these were carefully recorded in order to determine what factors might lead to cardiovascular disease. The result has revealed much about risk factors such as lipids, hypertension, smoking. The findings have become classic and uniquely respected for their accuracy and dependability.

Our Dietary Fats: The New Understanding of Cholesterol

The very word "fat" produces an emotional reaction in most of us —and obesity is regarded by many physicians as *the* major American health problem today, affecting as it does 30 to 40 percent of us. As the late Dr. John H. Knowles, president of the Rockefeller Foundation and one of our leading public health experts, once said to me: "There's plenty of evidence that obesity leads to everything from premature onset of diabetes to strokes and heart attacks."

Fats actually constitute a diverse group of organic compounds and are often spoken of as lipids. They are essential to life, for they provide your body's greatest energy reserve and are an essential part of cell membranes which are so vital to the functioning of every cell, tissue and organ in your body. Your body can synthesize or manufacture certain fats and remodel others from dietary fats (those you eat) to the needed kinds. Dietary fats, however, supply certain fatty acids and fat-soluble vitamins which your body cannot synthesize. These fats also transport such essential compounds throughout the body and assist in their absorption into the cells and tissues where they are needed.

Over the past quarter century, repeated studies have shown that hyperlipidemia (an excess of fats or lipids in the blood) is closely linked to atherosclerosis. The villain and chief offender of these lipids in the development of atherosclerosis and its most serious complications is cholesterol. The Framingham Study has found cholesterol the only one of these lipids to have any association with the production of strokes. Paradoxically, cholesterol is present in almost every one of our tissues and those of other animals as well.

However, the cholesterol present in the blood comes from two sources—those absorbed from the food we eat and those made by the body itself. Most body tissues can synthesize cholesterol, but the chief source of its manufacture is the liver. In our diet it is present only in the food from animal sources such as meat, eggs and dairy products.

The vital nature of this blood cholesterol level was revealed by the Framingham Study, which showed that in men under the age of fifty there is a distinct increase in the incidence of stroke with rising blood cholesterol levels. In a study of fifteen hundred men followed for ten years in the Chicago People's Gas Study, a similar relationship was shown. The ratio narrows as men live on into their fifties, and this did seem odd—particularly since blood levels of cholesterol do rise with age, reaching a peak in the fifties. The relationship between blood cholesterol levels and heart attacks is even closer than in stroke, but in both a change in the relationship seems to take place about this age.

However, a whole new concept has come into being during the past ten years as the lipoproteins have been brought into this picture. With the greater volume of heart (cardiac) disease and its deaths than of stroke, studies in the past have concentrated on the heart. But any study of cardiac disease or atherosclerosis is at least in good part translatable into the problem of stroke, for athero-sclerosis plays a major role in all cardiovascular diseases and is a most serious factor in strokes, while cardiac disease itself is a risk factor in CVAs.

Dr. William P. Castelli, Director of Laboratories at the Fra-mingham Study, explains this seeming discrepancy in the role of cholesterol at different ages: "Recent findings from the Framingham Heart Studies . . . show that in people over the age of fifty, total blood cholesterol no longer predicts who will get a heart attack. While this might suggest a new challenge to the cholesterol theory, a detailed study of our findings proves otherwise. It also reveals some startling new information about cholesterol metabolism and risk assessment made on the bases of blood lipids. Blood lipids are a powerful predictor of risk." And this same approach should hold as true for stroke and atherosclerosis as for heart attacks.

If you were to put fats or lipids directly into your blood, you would end up with something like Italian salad dressing in which oil or fat, and vinegar or water, are mixed together: shake it all up and the oil disperses through the liquid in the form of tiny droplets; let it stand and it separates out into two layers. To solve this problem, nature has put the lipids—and cholesterol in particular —into special packets so that it can be transported by the blood without separating out into layers.

After lipids have been absorbed by the intestines from food or manufactured by the liver, they have to be carried to those tissues in which the body will either burn them as fuel, utilize them to form cell membranes or simply store them in fatty tissues. In these packets the lipids—cholesterol, triglycerids and phospholipids— are combined with proteins to form what are called lipoproteins.

There are five major types of these packets, or lipoproteins, in our blood. Each contains a different percentage of the lipids and proteins, and they are classified in accordance with their density or weight—as chylomicrons (almost all triglyceride and lowest of all in density) through very-low-density lipoproteins (VLDL, with a lower percentage of triglyceride, more cholesterol and protein) and low-density lipoprotein (LDL) to high-density lipoprotein (HDL, with lower cholesterol and the largest percentage of protein of all).

The fats absorbed from the intestines are carried in the chylomicrons, while the VLDL is chiefly synthesized in the liver. Both of these forms may be converted to LDL, which transports a great deal of the cholesterol in your blood. The HDL also transports cholesterol, but here is where the amazing new knowledge has changed the picture. It has now been proved that while the LDLs are atherogenic (that is, produce atherosclerosis), a high level of HDL can actually protect against atherosclerosis.

We have already seen that in those under the age of fifty, high levels of cholesterol appear along with a higher incidence of stroke, while this connection is not nearly as strong in older people. As Dr. Castelli explains: "LDLs are predictors of risk in the same sense as the total cholesterol is in younger people; the higher it is, the worse it is. We know this kind of cholesterol is related to eating cholesterol and saturated fat. If you feed an animal too many foods rich in cholesterol and saturated fat, that animal's LDLs will begin to clog that animal's blood vessels and the animal will have either a heart attack or a stroke . . . We feel this same process goes on in humans. HDLs appear to oppose this process . . . to play a role in removing cholesterol from the body." The suspicion is that by blocking the uptake of cholesterol by body cells, HDLs actually interrupt or interfere with the basic process that produces atherosclerosis.

Lowering the Bad Cholesterol and Raising the Good: Diet and Exercise

We are born with roughly half our cholesterol in the form of HDLs, but the typical American diet tends to replace some of the HDLs with the more dangerous kind. The average cholesterol level for American men is 230 milligram percent in 100 milliliters (about one tenth of a quart) of blood—doctors simply say, "Your cholesterol is 230." Adult women have slightly lower levels. Men have an average HDL level of about 45 mg. percent, women about 55 —and some experts think this may be why women have less coronary heart disease. A Cincinnati research group studied a series of families known for consistently living into their eighties and nineties without serious cardiovascular disease and found extremely high HDL levels (usually 75 or more) among these people.

Thus, knowing a person's HDL level is thought important today in any assessment of the risk of cardiovascular disease. As we get older, the total blood cholesterol is now believed to have less value in predicting the risk, but the exact levels of cholesterol and LDLs and HDLs that are safest are still debatable. The Framingham Study found that in men between the ages of thirty and sixty-two, cholesterol levels of 250 carried about three times the risk of heart attack and stroke as did cholesterol levels under 194.

Dr. Robert Wissler, professor of pathology at the Chicago Pritzker School of Medicine, points out that "90 percent of the world's population have serum [blood] cholesterol levels of around 150 or lower and virtually never die of coronary occlusion [heart attacks]." He feels that the level American physicians consider "within the normal range"—up to 250—is probably too high. Other experts, too, talk of a similar cholesterol range—150 to 180 —as being the ideal: this is the level found among the Japanese, whose risk of coronary artery disease is one-eighth that of Americans with an average cholesterol level of around 230.

Experimental studies done on monkeys have produced atherosclerotic plaques in those animals fed high-fat, high-cholesterol diets. These plaques were then made to regress gradually when the animals were switched to diet and/or drug regimes which reduced their blood cholesterol levels down to 200 or less. NHLBI experts conclude: "This suggests that some stage of atherosclerosis can also be halted or reversed in humans, although this remains unproven."

An interesting study was made by a medical team at the University of Southern California School of Medicine which managed to achieve actual regression of early atherosclerotic plaques in the femoral (leg) arteries of nine patients who had excessive blood levels of either LDL or VLDL. This feat was accomplished by placing the patients on special NHLBI diets designed to lower such blood lipids, along with medication. The team succeeded in significantly reducing cholesterol, triglyceride and blood-pressure levels. These diets sharply limited the cholesterol and saturated fats eaten and greatly increased the polyunsaturated fats in the diet.

You probably have heard a good deal in recent years about diet and polyunsaturated fats. The distinction between saturated and unsaturated fats is a chemical one. A chain of carbon atoms makes up the backbone of these chemicals—when it has as many hydrogen atoms as it can hold it is termed saturated; when two hydrogen atoms can still be added it is called monounsaturated; and if there is room for four or more such atoms it is termed polyunsaturated. In some not yet understood way, polyunsaturated fats reduce cholesterol levels even if the individual continues eating food containing the same amount of cholesterol as before. On the other hand, saturated fats increase cholesterol levels and the monounsaturated ones have no influence.

Cholesterol-lowering diets require both expertise and a knowledge of your physical health and medical conditions. Before undertaking any changes in your diet, it is always best to consult your own physician because often simply reducing weight to normal limits is sufficient to reduce cholesterol to healthy levels. NHLBI experts suggest that to protect yourself against atherosclerosis and its complications, you might adopt what they term "prudent patterns of diet." And this, they advise, includes:

1. Regulating intake of calories so as to reach and maintain desirable body weight
2. Avoiding excessive intake of cholesterol (present in eggs, meat and dairy products) and of saturated (mainly animal) fats
3. Substituting, where possible, polyunsaturated fats (mainly from vegetable or marine oils) for saturated fats
4. Keeping salt intake within reasonable limits

There are special diets available from NHLBI for those with particular medical problems such as excessive blood-lipid levels due to hereditary or dietary causes. Another useful and authoritative source is *The American Heart Association Cookbook,* which provides information on the amounts of total fat and cholesterol you should have in your diet, and the levels of saturated and polyunsaturated fats, along with charts listing the amounts of these elements in a wide range of meats, fish, dairy products and margarines.

Interestingly, it has been shown that HDL is high in cross-country skiers and marathon runners, and it can also be raised with very moderate physical activity. For example, in a recent study at

Canada's University of Manitoba, men with coronary artery disease were put on a thirteen-week program of walking or slow jogging twenty to thirty minutes, three times a week, for little more than a mile and a half, yet the HDL levels of these people promptly rose. Only time can tell whether this will truly have a protective effect.

Children and Cholesterol

One study has shown that 20 percent of young people, aged fifteen to twenty, had coronary artery atherosclerosis. Other studies have revealed that 77 percent of our soldiers who died in the Korean War and 45 percent of those killed in the Vietnam conflict had similar evidences of atherosclerosis at an average age of twenty-two. Obviously, if we are to protect our children, we must start in early childhood.

The American Heart Association recently came out with an official statement issued for physician's guidance—and one from which parents can learn. It recommended that children in families with a high risk of cardiovascular disease be examined by a physician and placed on a corrective diet if they show excessive blood-lipid levels. A high-risk family is considered to be one in which either or both parents have hyperlipidemia or hypertension—or in which parents or grandparents have suffered a heart attack or stroke or have had peripheral vascular disease (atherosclerosis, usually in the extremities) before the age of fifty.

This statement also added that "although the evidence does not yet support the recommendation that cholesterol and saturated fat should be reduced in the diet of all children, the public should be advised that such modification appears safe and very likely to be beneficial in reducing or retarding the risk of atherosclerotic disease in their adult years."

The American Heart Association advises that children from high-risk families should be carefully checked for hyperlipidemia with "at least two, preferably three, repetitive samplings" of blood fats, and medical opinion is nearly unanimous about the need to change the diet of such children. Recent surveys have shown conclusively that American children have higher blood-lipid levels than children in other countries have. In fact, about 5 percent of our youngsters from five to eighteen years of age have cholesterol levels over 200 to 220. As American Heart experts explain: "Because hyperlipidemia is the most consistent and frequent risk factor for atherosclerotic disease (other than age and sex), it has received the most attention as a point of attack for the prevention of atherosclerosis."

Helping Yourself to Prevention: The Risk Factors

As NHLBI experts put it: "Some risk factors are more definitely associated with the development of coronary heart disease, stroke, and peripheral artery disease than others." By familiarizing yourself with these risk factors you can readily identify those which may apply to you and take the necessary steps—with or without the help of your physician—to protect yourself against or even to eliminate these as far as possible. These experts divide the risk factors into three categories, although the differences between the categories are at times a matter of rather fine distinctions:

I. The Established Risk Factors:
1. High concentrations of blood cholesterol
2. High blood pressure
3. Cigarette smoking

II. Probable Risk Factors
1. Diabetes
2. Stress and coronary-prone behavior
3. Postmenopausal state
4. Family history and genetic factors
5. Contraceptive pills

III. Suspected Risk Factors
1. Overweight
2. Physical inactivity

We have discussed the problem of high blood cholesterol levels at sufficient length—but you can seen how NHLBI experts regard this problem as a first priority. Your physician can measure its levels with a simple blood test.

High blood pressure, or hypertension, is so directly tied to stroke that the risk of a CVA rises directly with the increasing level of hypertension. So important and complex is this problem that we will devote our next chapter to it.

Cigarette smoking strikes in several ways. The Framingham Study has indicated that cigarette smoking triples the risk of cerebral infarction. Recently the study has also identified an actual drop in the protective HDLs in both men and women: the more they smoked, the greater this drop. Moreover, cigarettes are proved to be associated with an increased risk of coronary artery disease, which itself is associated with an increased risk of stroke. And smoking is a major factor in those strokes resulting from the use of oral contraceptives (see below).

Diabetes is often associated with hyperlipidemia, hypertension and obestity. However, the experts at NHLBI feel that these problems—all of which are themselves associated with a higher risk of stroke—cannot of themselves explain the entire increase in stroke found among diabetics. Regular medical checkups are the key to finding diabetes early—and careful adherence to the medical regimen prescribed for the disease is vital if the added risk of stroke is to be limited as far as possible.

Stress is suspect in the development of both atherosclerosis and of stroke. However, the coronary-prone so-called "Type A" behavior pattern will increase the risk of stroke. Drs. Meyer Friedman and Ray H. Rosenman, the San Francisco cardiologists who developed this hypothesis of Type A behavior as characteristic of most heart-attack victims, observed a group of accountants during their tense time-pressured tax season and found that both cholesterol levels and blood-clotting rates rose from January to the April 15 tax deadline—and both of these are risk factors for strokes.

The postmenopausal state carries with it the fact that the woman is getting older and age is a definite factor in the incidence of stroke. However, there are indications that the menopause (natural or surgically induced) carries with it a greater risk of cardiovascular disease, so the menopausal and postmenopausal woman should adhere to a pattern of regular medical examinations and follow medical advice. The menopause also brings increased coronary heart disease, and this too increases the risk of stroke. In fact, premenopausal women have significantly less, and less severe, coronary heart disease than women of the same age with surgically induced menopause.

The role of family history and genetic factors in stroke are not entirely clear. While some families do show a history of premature heart attacks, it is uncertain whether this is due to genetic factors, the sharing of a similar lifestyle, environment and dietary habits. There is evidence that some forms of hyperlipidemia, hypertension and diabetes may have a genetic component—and all these are definite risk factors in stroke. The person with such a family history should be doubly careful—make certain his doctor is aware of this, faithfully follow regular medical checkups and the physician's instructions.

Contraceptive pills are a very serious problem today. One extensive study carried out in the United Kingdom by the Royal College of General Practitioners revealed that the death rate from cardiovascular diseases in women using oral contraceptives was five times that of those who had never used them, and the death rate in those taking the pill continuously for five years or more was ten times that of others due to cardiovascular diseases. Excessive death rate increased with age, cigarette smoking and the duration of contraceptive use.

So serious is this combination of oral contraceptive and cigarette smoking that Dr. Savitri Ramcharan, Kaiser-Permanente Contraceptive Drug Study, Walnut Creek, California, says: "Smoking should be considered a contraindication to oral-contraceptive use, or at the very least, women wishing to use oral contraceptives should be strongly urged not to smoke."

In this study of nearly seventeen thousand women for more than six years, the team of investigators from Kaiser-Permanente and the U.S. Center for Disease Control in Atlanta found (like others before it) that the use of oral contraceptives sharply increased the

chance of both vascular disease and stroke. And smoking significantly increased the risk of stroke—add the two (smoking and the
pill) together and the result is disaster. The study also showed a
sharp increase in stroke with smoking alone. Among these women,
hemorrhagic strokes were 5.7 times as common among the smokers
as among the nonsmokers, and other strokes were 4.8 times as
common. But among the oral-contraceptive users who also
smoked, this risk figure skyrocketed to 21.9!

Obesity, too, definitely increases the risk of stroke. The NHLBI
scientists feel that much of this effect occurs through the other risk
factors with which obesity is commonly associated—hyperlipidemia, hypertension and diabetes. Moreover, obese individuals
usually have lower levels of HDL and are less active physically. In
a University of Michigan School of Medicine study, Dr. Allen B.
Nichols and his colleagues found that hyperlipidemia was much
more related to the degree of obesity than the particular diet being
consumed. In fact, Dr. Nichols concludes: "From the findings in
this study, one may infer that weight reduction should be the initial
intervention for control of hyperlipidemia in the general population."

7

THE CAUSES OF STROKES AND HOW TO PROTECT YOURSELF (PART 2):

Hypertension, the Silent Killer; Self-Care and Prevention

It doesn't make the room whirl about you nor does it throb like a toothache—which is unfortunate because if it did, two thirds to three quarters of those who have suffered strokes in their fifties and sixties might have avoided them. And four fifths of those would have escaped dying as and when they did, for we don't let toothaches go unattended—severe discomforts are taken care of promptly. There is no such disease as "high blood pressure" any more than there is any such disease as "hyperthermia" (high fever), for these are only symptoms, disorders, conditions and not diseases. Hypertension is a symptom of something going wrong with the bodily processes or health.

The Framingham Study found hypertension to be two to seventeen times as great a contributor to stroke as any other risk factor. From their eighteen-year follow-up, Framingham Study experts conclude that in the development of atherosclerotic and thrombotic brain infarction, "hypertension is the most common and most powerful precursor." These CVAs struck hypertensive patients seven times more often than it did those with normal pressure, and summing up this situation, these experts said that "the risk was proportional to the blood pressure throughout its range." In short, the higher the blood pressure, the greater the risk. Hypertensive patients suffered these strokes "at from five to more than thirty times the rate of normotensive persons [those with normal blood pressure]."

Here, in this world of hypertension, Americans must act personally and positively to vastly reduce the risk of suffering strokes, to prevent them in many instances. Here, too, parents have an opportunity to protect their children from suffering a CVA in adult life. Since hypertension has its roots in the very first years of life, blood pressure should be checked regularly from the child's second birthday on.

Perhaps the most shocking aspect of hypertension lies in the fact that it can have so tragic an outcome yet is so often neglected, even though its detection is quick, painless and simple, its treatment typically only a matter of pill taking and proper diet. A recent report of a Mayo Clinic three-community study surprised all observers by revealing that 60 percent of adults who knew they had hypertension still failed either to accept treatment for it or to continue the therapeutic measures once they were prescribed for them.

The importance of this condition comes not only from the tragic consequences if it is neglected (either in having it diagnosed or in not following the prescribed care) but from the large number of Americans involved. According to the very latest (1979) figures of the National Institutes of Health's new arm, the National High Blood Pressure Education Program (NHBPEP, established in the early 1970s), thirty-five million Americans have definite hypertension and need ongoing treatment, while another twenty-five million are estimated to have "borderline" hypertension which calls for regular medical supervision.

In the words of NHBPEP experts: "These very nearly sixty million American adults face the increased risk of heart attack, stroke, and kidney failure because of elevated blood pressure. The disease is more common among blacks than whites—about one out of four blacks has definite hypertension, compared to about one out of six in the total population."

These problems are not limited to the United States, as a twelve-nation hypertension meeting at the World Health Organization (WHO) in Geneva in 1978 proved. The major generalization agreed upon by these experts from around the world was that hypertension is directly related to so-called civilization. What has become quite clear is that hypertension is truly the chief epidemic of our twentieth century; WHO estimates that hypertension today afflicts 20 percent of the entire world's middle-aged people!

The problem is now so acute that WHO devoted its 1978 World Health Day to "Down With High Blood Pressure," although the disorder does vary geographically in degree. In Japan, for example, stroke comprises 25 percent of the annual death rate, and in especially stroke-prone communities there, 80 percent of those who die from stroke have suffered from hypertension. In China, where stroke is second only to all cardiovascular diseases as a cause of death, hypertension is widespread. In Russia, the head of Moscow's Institute of Cardiology has become actively involved in utilizing radio and TV appearances to attempt to get to his countrymen the same messages about hypertension that our NHBPEP seeks to spread here. And in Cuba, 90 percent of heart-disease patients have hypertension.

Here in the United States, too, hypertension is one of our worst health problems. Dr. William Hollander, professor of medicine at Boston University, points out that hypertension in America is a major cause of one quarter to one half of all our cardiovascular deaths. And while there is no cure for hypertension, it can most certainly be controlled. According to Dr. Hollander, it is possible today to provide "almost complete protection against strokes" by early treatment of hypertension. Many experts believe that it is our more effective management of hypertension that is the major factor in the recent drop in both stroke and heart disease—and has added three years to the life expectancy of Americans, men and women, whites and blacks.

But the ultimate success of this control of hypertension depends entirely on the public—on whether they will join in finding out whether they themselves are hypertensives, and if so, cooperate in the treatment of their own problem. For this, however, you need to know a number of things about blood pressure: what it is, what is normal and abnormal; what is excessive and what causes it to become this way; what harm hypertension can do and whether it is curable or correctible; what the varied kinds are and the special problems of children and teen-agers and how to protect them; the values and dangers of exercise, of salt, diet and obesity, and even those of the Pill.

What *Is* Blood Pressure?

The circulatory system of your body is actually a major transportation system that has the responsibility for seeing to it that five quarts of a rather sluggish fluid are kept moving constantly through more than sixty thousand miles of blood vessels, many only microscopic in size. The red blood cells carried in this fluid can barely get through the smaller tubes, the capillaries, even in single file. Yet both cells and fluid must be delivered constantly to an estimated one hundred trillion body cells, some of which will be permanently or even fatally injured should delivery of the blood and its contents be held up for as little as five minutes or so. It requires no thinking, since it's a completely automatic system, both self-operated and self-correcting. Thus it's not surprising that things do go wrong sometimes—perhaps it's even more astonishing that things go wrong so rarely.

To drive the blood through the sixty thousand miles of vessels to every part of your body (straight uphill when you're standing) obviously requires an immensely powerful and hard-working pump—and a long-lasting one, for it must operate every minute of every day of your life. This is the task set your heart, a fist-sized muscle which contracts, or "beats," seventy times a minute (automatically speeding up when you exercise or eat or get excited)—thirty-six million times a year. By the time you are fifty years old, this formidable organ will have beat two billion times and pumped more than three hundred thousand tons of blood.

Your heart is actually a four-chambered pump, blood coming into the top two chambers (the atria) and being pumped out of the bottom two (the ventricles). This organ could in fact be considered two pumps. The blood coming back from the body flows into the right side of the heart and is then sent to the lungs to get rid of its gases (essentially carbon dioxide), load up with oxygen and then return to the left side of the heart, from which it is pumped into the aorta, your body's largest and chief artery. From the aorta the blood is driven through ever smaller arteries as these divide and subdivide until they become arterioles, narrow arteries with muscular coats which are under automatic-nervous-system control.

The arterioles keep the blood from flooding the capillaries, which are barely wide enough for a red blood cell to slip through. The walls of the capillaries are thin (one cell thick), so that through them nutrients and oxygen diffuse to feed the tissues of your body, and cellular wastes are discharged. From here the blood moves on into venules, or tiny veins, and then ever larger veins as the blood retraces its way back to your heart.

The arterioles see to it too that your tissues get enough blood. During exercise your muscles need more blood, so the arterioles automatically dilate—as do those of stomach and intestines during eating and digestion. It's the task of the arterioles to also make certain that your brain gets enough blood. When you're standing, the arterioles of the legs constrict so that more blood is available for the brain instead of accumulating in the legs. By such vascular action the blood is shunted around your body to where it is most needed at any particular time.

Blood pressure is actually the pressure of the blood as it presses against the walls of the arteries it flows through. But it is essentially the arterioles that determine this pressure. Imagine a rubber hose connected to a faucet whose valve is turned on: the narrower the hose or the opening of the hose nozzle, the greater the pressure of the water at the faucet. To look at this another way: were you to make the hose nozzle opening smaller, the hose would harden or even bulge out behind the nozzle as the pressure builds up in the hose and against its walls (or those of an artery should its arterioles narrow down as its muscles contract). Most hypertension is believed to be related in some way to faulty functioning of the arterioles.

The blood is pumped out of your heart by a simple squeezing

action of its muscle. It's not unlike holding in the palm of your hand a rubber bulb syringe with a nozzle, all filled with water; simply squeezing down hard on the bulb expels all the water. When the heart contracts and drives the blood into the arterial system, this is called systole—and the blood pressure that then results is called systolic pressure.

If the nozzle of the squeezed bulb were now placed in a pan of water and the bulb released, it would expand and get filled with water—just as your heart muscle relaxes after systole and the ventricles fill once more with blood. This is called diastole—and the blood pressure at this time is termed diastolic pressure. Incidentally, in systole the heart actually forces out roughly half a cup of blood into the aorta. Systole (so called from the Greek word for "contraction") lasts less than half a second, and diastole (Greek for "dilation") perhaps a trifle more.

There is a marked rise in blood pressure during systole, the power phase, and systolic pressure is high because the ventricles are forcing blood into the arterial system. When this pressure stops during diastole, the blood pressure drops as the wave of blood flows through arteries, arterioles, capillaries and venous system to fill the heart from the top and prepare the way for the systolic phase, the pumping of the next spurt of blood from the heart. You can feel this rise and fall of pressure in your own arteries if you feel the "pulse" in your wrist (as doctors do to tell the pace of your heart, how many beats per minute).

Measuring Blood Pressure

This is a simple, painless procedure—so much so that doctors often teach patients to do it themselves. The device used is something called a sphygmomanometer (from the Greek *sphygmós,* meaning pulse), invented almost a hundred years ago by a noted French heart specialist, Pierre Carl Edouard Potain. The instrument is based on the principle that if you put mercury into a U-shaped glass tube and pump air into the top of one arm of the U, the mercury will rise in the other arm to a level which will depend on the air pressure. If you put a gauge in millimeters (mm.) alongside one arm, you can then measure in mm. of mercury the amount of air pressure being pumped.

Your doctor uses his sphygmomanometer by wrapping an inflatable cloth cuff around your arm just above the elbow. This cuff is connected to the column of mercury in the instrument by one tube, and by another to a simple rubber bulb. First the physician squeezes the bulb and inflates the cuff so that he drives the mercury column up to near the top of its gauge, or scale. The resulting air pressure in the cuff compresses your large brachial (upper-arm) artery to the point where the pressure of the blood flow is no longer strong enough to force its way past this pressure obstruction, this compression.

The physician now places a stethoscope over the artery just below the cuff. Since at this point no blood can flow to the forearm, there is no sound in the artery. As the pressure is gradually reduced when some of the air in the cuff is allowed to slowly escape, the column of mercury falls. Watching this column carefully while still listening, the physician continues to release air until the pressure of the blood—your blood pressure—is finally equal to that of the air in the cuff.

At this point the blood flow through the artery finally resumes, and the doctor hears a thudding sort of sound in the stethoscope. The reading in mm. on the mercury gauge is now recorded; this indicates your greatest blood pressure—when the heart contracts —and this is the systolic pressure.

Your doctor continues to release air very slowly and gradually. With the first overcoming of the cuff's pressure the thudding sound is faint, but then it grows stronger as the blood pulses through the artery. But then it begins to fade and eventually once more becomes discernible. Again your doctor carefully notes the reading on the mercury gauge—this time when the sound is last detected. This is the lowest level of your blood pressure and occurs when your heart has relaxed between its contractions, its beats—this is the diastolic pressure.

Your doctor will then record the two pressures on your chart as a pair of numbers with a slash between. For a blood pressure reading that is considered fairly normal for an adult between the ages of eighteen and forty-five this would be written 120/80. Or if you asked your doctor what it was he would simply say, "Your blood pressure is 120 over 80"—which means that your systolic pressure is 120 mm. of mercury, and your diastolic is 80 mm.

Normal Blood Pressure and Hypertension—The Kinds and the Numbers

While it is an easy and uncontroversial matter to say that arterial blood pressure of 120 systolic and 80 diastolic—120/80—is normal from the age of eighteen on, or that 250/150 is abnormal regardless of age, it is in the intermediate ranges—say, around 140/90 or 145/95—that definitions become rather arbitrary and controversial. Take the middle-aged man whose blood pressure has always been 120/80 and on a checkup finds that it's 140/85. Alarmed, he wants to know if he has hypertension. However, by the time he is ready to leave, his pressure is back to 120/80. He had been tense that morning and hurried, was worried about his examination—so his blood pressure went up.

Fortunately, your arterial walls are quite elastic. Were it not for this, the blood pressure within them would become intolerably high in systole as the heart pumps blood into them. But when the heart relaxes in diastole, the pressure would quickly drop to zero, and there would be no blood flowing through the capillaries because the arteries have to be able to constrict and narrow to maintain the necessary pressure during diastole. Thus the arterial system, which normally operates automatically to dampen and restrict the pressure, swings up and down during the heart's cycle of systole-diastole.

In fact, the importance of this elasticity in keeping blood pressure within acceptable body limits is made clear by a common problem that arises with advancing years. The elasticity of the larger arteries inexorably decreases as we grow older, resulting in what doctors term systolic hypertension. With increasing age the larger arteries can become almost as rigid as your garden hose, and with this condition, the systolic pressure can rise to 160, 180, even 200, while the diastolic drops to 60, 50 and even less.

The area of blood pressure today tends to be a sort of numbers game with changing figures and definitions that are imprecise at best. The extremes are perfectly clear, and blood-pressure determinations can be made quite accurately. But what the figures mean —which ones should be treated as indications of hypertension and which not—is being hotly debated as doctors have become aware as never before of the dangers of hypertension. And yet an enormous part of the hypertensive public is going untreated and at serious risk of a shortened or crippled life.

Blood pressure varies considerably in a person from day to day and even from minute to minute. It goes up when you are under stress at the office or watching an exciting football game on TV, indulging in a passionate kiss, playing tennis or bridge. By simply breathing deeply for a minute or two or relaxing fully, some people can drop their pressure by as much as twenty or thirty points, which is why doctors will always use several pressure measurements before deciding that a patient has high or low pressure. Some people have sudden spurts of high blood pressure—the reason why you see someone "getting red in the face" when angry, or the blood pounding in his temples.

A belief of an earlier and somewhat more naïve medical day held that your normal systolic pressure was 100 plus your age—but this is now known to be wrong. But what is abnormal tension? First, it must be a reading that stays at a higher figure consistently, but what this figure should be is still a source of debate. Some physicians feel that only when the pressure goes up to 140/90 consistently is there any need for intervention, while others won't start any treatment before 150/90 or even 160/90.

It was only a decade ago that diastolic pressure was considered by far the more important of the two measurements, with systolic being regarded as not nearly as significant. But today, as Dr. Irvine H. Page, famous pioneer and cardiovascular expert of the Cleveland Clinic, points out: "It has recently become modish to proclaim that systolic pressure is a better guide to prognosis than the diastolic." Moreover, the systolic pressure is now thought to correlate more closely with vascular problems—and especially stroke. But Dr. Page recalls seeing blood pressure measured at thirty-second intervals changing from 156/92 to 148/88, then to 140/86 and finally 133/84. Looking at just one figure, the person could be considered hypertensive, borderline hypertensive or normal—yet the changes all happened within seconds, showing how labile pressure is.

It's hard to find broadly acceptable and precise definitions. Experts at the Mayo Clinic, for example, define borderline hypertension as pressures between 140/90 and 159/94. Hypertension they define as "sustained blood pressure readings greater than 160/95." But there are many experts who define mild hypertension as a range of systolic readings from 140 to 160 with the diastolic from 90 to 110. In severe hypertension the blood pressure can go as high as 200/115. In the most dangerous type—malignant or accelerating hypertension—it can even go as high as 240/150. One expert highlights this confusion by referring to mild hypertension as a euphemism for those pressures which doctors don't know whether to treat or not.

Dr. W. McFate Smith, University of California/San Francisco professor of medicine, sums up the issue: "There is no single level of blood pressure which seperates normotensives from hypertensives, nor 'milds' from more severe hypertensives." He emphasizes "the wide variability, within individuals, of pressure levels on successive measurements . . . The members of a given blood pressure class are not entirely the same at different points in time." Which is why the public must beware of the machines for taking their pressure found today in a wide variety of public facilities, for it is the interpretation of this figure which is so important, and so difficult.

Hypertension: The Symptoms—The Causes—Those at Risk

Hypertension is insidious because it has no characteristic warning symptoms and usually has none at all. True, hypertensives may have headaches, usually at the back of the head or upper part of the neck, that may appear on awakening in the early morning. But such headaches are common among those without hypertension and due to a host of other reasons. Dizziness or light-headedness may also trouble hypertensives, but these symptoms too may indicate other disorders.

At least nine out of ten hypertensives suffer from what doctors term essential, or idiopathic, hypertension, meaning that the cause is unknown. However, heredity is an important factor, which has been shown in a number of ways. Essential hypertension appears more often in those with a family history of this disorder: if one parent suffers from this condition, there is a 50 percent chance that the children will develop it (usually in their forties); if both parents have the problem, the chance of a child having it is 90 percent. The role of heredity in hypertension has been shown in such studies as those of twins: the blood pressure of identical twins is much closer to each other than that of nonidentical twins (whose genes are not exactly the same).

Although the cause of essential hypertension is unknown, there are certain factors known to aggravate it: stress and emotional tension, ingesting too much salt, cigarette smoking and obesity.

The other kind of hypertension—secondary hypertension—includes those conditions due to ascertainable and definite known causes. For example, it may be due to atherosclerosis or kidney disorders, hormonal disturbances (as adrenal overactivity), pregnancy, and the like.

Hypertension, like stroke itself, becomes increasingly common with age, although it too can happen at any time in life and to any person. Men seem at greater risk, for it strikes them more often and in more severe form than women. Blacks suffer almost twice as high a rate of this disorder; and their death rates are from three to twelve times as high, and most often from stroke. Oral contraceptives—the Pill—also seems to put women at risk of hypertension and many experts urge careful regular blood-pressure checks when a woman starts taking the Pill for the first time. Pregnancy, too, may put women at risk of hypertension.

It has been found that not only obese people but also those who are bigger physically are in greater danger of developing hypertension. An international team of medical scientists found that South Americans living in the mountains have lower blood pressure than their countrymen at the seashore—because those in the mountains are smaller in size. And among civil service workers in Israel a study found that overweight is "the one outstanding precursor of hypertension with an impact apparently overshadowing that of age."

Hypertension: Its Effects and Its Treatment

Dr. Marvin Moser, professor of medicine at New York Medical College, spells it out precisely: "Approximately 85 percent of strokes are the result of hypertension in patients in their fifties and sixties, and about 60 to 75 percent of these can probably be prevented with control of the hypertension. Recurrent strokes can also be prevented by appropriate blood-pressure-lowering."

Hypertension attacks the blood vessels, damaging both large and small arteries as well as arterioles. The high pressure produces atherosclerosis, or accelerates any already present. For some reason this atherosclerosis from hypertension has a particular affinity for the tiny arteries serving brain and heart. But even without atherosclerosis, the walls of the arteries thicken and their lumen is narrowed by this elevated pressure.

Heightened blood pressure also produces other effects. It can injure the intima of the arteries which initiates an atherosclerotic process or thrombus formation or both, and from this can come the emboli which are such major causes of strokes. Finally, too, the elevated pressure can rupture any weakened artery in the brain— whether caused by an aneurysm or an atherosclerotic plaque—and so lead to a hemorrhagic stroke.

"Strokes rarely occur in well-treated hypertensive patients under the age of seventy," Dr. Moser explains. "Recurrent strokes can also be prevented by appropriate blood-pressure-lowering."

As we have already seen, except for those rare secondary strokes whose cause is known and therefore can be treated, the only cause of stroke that can be treated and relieved is really hypertension.

And while hypertension cannot be cured, it can be controlled, and experts today feel that this is the most important thing in preventing its complications. In fact, experimental studies at Boston University School of Medicine have shown that when hypertension is controlled soon after its onset, strokes due to atherosclerosis or cerebral vessel ruptures are almost entirely prevented!

Obviously the first step is diagnosis, and this can only be accomplished by regular medical checkups, since there are no distinctive symptoms of hypertension. But once the problem has been diagnosed with the simple blood-pressure test, your doctor has at his command a number of tools for reducing high blood pressure and keeping it that way. The attack is multidimensional. Some cases of essential hypertension can be controlled with simple changes in life style: relieving emotional tension by increased relaxation and exercise, bringing weight down to normal and reducing salt intake. When any or all of this does not help, doctors have a vast array of drugs available today. Should the problem prove to be secondary hypertension, it becomes a matter of diagnosing the cause and treating this (kidney disturbances, hormonal imbalances, and the like).

That medication works for hypertension—and prevents strokes —is a proven fact. In two major studies by the Veterans Administration Cooperative Study involving some fifteen VA hospitals across the nation, the results were striking and entirely conclusive: the risk of developing complications from hypertension in those with diastolic pressure of 90 to 114 were reduced in a five-year period from 55 percent in those who received only placebos (sugar pills) to 18 percent in those given antihypertensive medication, with thirty-five dying in the placebo group to only nine under active treatment. The chief benefits of this antihypertensive therapy proved to be the prevention of stroke and heart failure. In another study of patients with 115 to 129 diastolic pressure, the results were equally dramatic, with a 50 percent reduction in mortality and a two-thirds reduction in morbidity and mortality among the treated group—and here again the prevention of strokes was the primary benefit.

So those with hypertension today can anticipate what one expert terms "overwhelming" benefits from treatment. Three classes of drugs form the backbone and mainstay of antihypertensive therapy. First are the diuretics (the "water pills") which promote excretion of salt and water from the body. Actually, the diuretics alone can reduce arterial pressure by as much as 10 to 15 percent. In addition, they increase the efficacy of other drugs, so they are often prescribed in combination with other medication.

The second class of drugs used are the vasodilators, which relax the muscles in the wall of arteries and veins. This type of drug enlarges the channels through which the blood flows and thus reduces the pressure, as opening the nozzle on a water hose does.

The third and last category are the drugs that inhibit the nervous system controlling the musculature of the blood-vessel walls. These drugs may either relax the blood vessels or slow down the heart (sometimes the hypertensive's heart rate is so fast that it serves to raise the pressure) and reduce the force of its contractions.

Occasionally, as with all powerful drugs, there may be side effects such as general weakness, rapid forceful heartbeat, stomach or intestinal upsets, or even sexual disorders. But if the patient reports these promptly to his doctor and changes are made either in the drug used or in its dosage, the side effects can be reduced or entirely eliminated. Moreover, as time goes on, these drugs are being steadily improved, and new and more effective ones with fewer side effects are introduced—so if you had difficulties in the past, these may well be resolved in the future. Experts feel the outlook for improving such medication is better than it has ever been.

The entire success of any treatment depends on the hypertensive's willingness to follow his doctor's prescribed regimen. Tragically, as the Mayo study demonstrated so dramatically, patient compliance with prescribed hypertensive care is not good. The hypertensive must, however, face up to his own responsibility here. He should make sure that he has a physician to whom he can relate well because this will help him feel comfortable and follow instructions in what has to be a long and ongoing relationship, since hypertension, like diabetes, usually means a lifetime of control.

Self-Care for Hypertensives

Dr. Ralph S. Paffenbarger, Stanford University epidemiologist, and his colleagues followed nearly fifteen thousand Harvard alumni aged thirty-five to seventy-four over a ten-year period. The results spell out how much you can do to reduce your own danger of hypertension, along with the strokes it threatens:

1. Men who took no vigorous exercise (swimming, running, tennis) were at 35 percent higher risk of hypertension than those who did.
2. Men who were 20 percent heavier than their ideal weight were at 78 percent greater risk of hypertension than leaner ones.
3. Men whose parents were hypertensive had 83 percent higher risk of getting the disease than those whose parents weren't.

You can do something about all these risk factors—even about your heredity. For those with this heredity can see to it that they get regular medical care, reduce other risk factors and follow their doctor's orders precisely.

In a carefully controlled Israeli study, nearly a hundred mildly hypertensive overweight patients were put on a weight-reducing program. In six months these Israelis lost an average of twenty-three pounds—and their tension dropped an average of 25/20, so that two-thirds now had normal tension.

Excessive salt intake is another problem that concerns the experts. A number of studies have already shown that fewer salty foods and a reduction of the salt in cooking and on food during meals—cutting in half the amount of salt previously ingested—can produce an average drop of 10 mm. in blood pressure.

Exercise, many experts believe, is also of considerable help in controlling hypertension. But Dr. Sidney Blumenthal, formerly director of the NHLBI Division of Heart and Vascular Diseases and now special assistant to the NHLBI director, warns that "certain kinds of exercise raise blood pressure, while others do not. Rhythmic exercises do not and are healthy—walking, running, golf, baseball. But the static exercises—wrestling or weight lifting are classic examples—very much raise the blood pressure." In short, there are "good" and "bad" exercises: the isometric exercises such as weight lifting rank among the "bad" ones.

Such experts seem to agree that the new techniques which have become popular in recent years for inducing relaxation—biofeedback, transcendental meditation, and the like—seem to lower blood pressure in some patients. But just how this comes about is unclear at this time—nor is there any certainty about how long such an effect will last.

How to Protect Children and Adolescents

As Dr. Blumenthal points out: "There is general acceptance of the concept that hypertension in the adult has its roots in childhood." And Dr. Lot B. Page, professor of medicine at Tufts University, urges parents and doctors alike: "If we can change the American dietary pattern in infancy, we can prevent high blood pressure. Even though heredity is a major determinant . . . two other factors are required to actually induce it. One is high salt intake. The other is obesity."

On the usual American diet, the child of hypertensive parents can have a slightly raised blood pressure by the age of two. Dr. Page points out that parents can prevent hypertension by "not letting our infants and young children develop the taste for salt, which becomes as addictive as smoking." If rats that are genetically susceptible to hypertension are never given salt, their tension remains normal throughout life, but if given salt when they are young, they eventually develop hypertension even if salt is later stopped.

Dr. Page also studied primitive societies. In eight Solomon Island preindustrial societies which have changed but little from primitive times, there was no hypertension until some members began to use salt and developed this problem. In eighteen societies free from hypertension, not one uses salt in its diet. But our American youngsters consume an enormous amount of salt—thanks to their hamburgers, pizzas, French fries, canned soups, bacon and cold cuts, cheese, snack chips, and the like. One specialist even asks: "Are we poisoning our children with salt?"

Experts all agree that checking blood pressure should be a routine part of the regular physical examination given children over the age of two. These physicians would be concerned if a child's blood pressure was at or above the 95th percentile (the top 5 percent) for his age, and doctors have tables showing such figures. For example, among three-year-olds, half will have blood pressure no higher than 95/64, while only 5 percent will have 112/80 or more; by the age of ten this will have risen to 110/70 and 130/92, respectively; and by the age of fifteen to 116/70 and 138/95. As more is learned, the figures for children are being revised to provide better bases for judging them. There are no major differences between girls and boys in this respect.

The prudent doctor does not depend on any single pressure-taking for a diagnosis of hypertension in youngsters but will insist on three separate readings. After the initial test he should take another a week later, and then one four or five weeks after that—which is what Dr. Blumenthal suggests.

The NHLBI expert points out that all youngsters in this top 5 percent of pressure readings should be under careful medical surveillance which, as he explains, "includes periodic examinations with blood pressure taken, avoidance of overweight, a very active physical-activity program, avoidance of salt abuse—and probably as important as any of these is avoidance of cigarette smoking or abstaining from developing the habit."

Youngsters with a family history of hypertension and premature heart attacks or strokes (those occurring before the age of fifty) in parents or grandparents are in a very special category. The handling of hypertension in youngsters is a highly specialized affair because there must be a decision on whether and when to go with diet, exercise and the rest of the non-drug therapies or to turn to the use of the antihypertensive medication. For exercise, Dr. Blumenthal says of the hypertensive child: "I would like to see him play baseball or basketball or golf or track or walk . . . but I would *not* like him to go out for the wrestling team or be a weight lifter."

On the use of medication for youngsters, this expert warns: "We think medication needs to be used with great care and then only under the supervision of a physician who has a lot of expertise in this field because we don't know what the side effects are of each of the medications in the youngster. When blood pressure is very high, here we think medication will probably be necessary but should only be used by someone who knows this field very well. It is different from adult medicine, but if a parent calls the local hospital and particularly the teaching center, they can tell the parent who in their institution or in the geographical area has a special interest in this problem in youngsters."

So hypertensive parents, or those whose own parents were hypertensive, should be especially aware that their child is at risk. Another group at special risk are black youngsters, and their parents should be very aware of this. As Br. Blumenthal explains: "The difference in blood pressure between blacks and whites makes its appearance at around fourteen or fifteen years of age—the black adolescent has a higher blood pressure than the white, and there is a small group of black adolescents who develop a very fulminating hypertension not seen in white children and we don't know why. Those black youngsters with this kind of blood-pressure rise can develop strokes, and we know why and don't understand it."

The widespread use of oral contraceptives by adolescents today is of concern, as Dr. Blumenthal also warns: "The Pill is a very important problem because of its effect on blood pressure. Any girl on the Pill should have her blood pressure taken regularly. When first on it, her blood pressure should be taken once a month for four or five months, and after that once a year—and the same is true of checking her blood level of triglycerides because the Pill will elevate these too. You can get a good lead on those who are going to get into trouble by knowing if there is a history of essential hypertension or elevated triglycerides in the family."

This NHLBI expert sums up his own feelings about this question: "I'm inherently opposed to the Pill—but not because I'm old-fashioned. I have two grown daughters and I have urged them to use some other contraceptive measures because the Pill has very real side effects, the same dangers as in the adults. The difference is that adolescents are pretty independent people and so much less apt to have close medical supervision because of the nature of adolescence. I feel very strongly that any girl on the Pill should have close medical supervision particularly during the first six months."

From the causes of stroke it is only logical that we should move to its treatment.

III

THE MODERN TREATMENT AND PREVENTION OF STROKE

8

THE MEDICAL ATTACK ON STROKE

What Happens; Its
Treatment;
the New Miracle Preventive;
the Blood and Its Role;
Stress

Like many others, a retired sixty-four-year-old New York businessman awoke one morning with slurred speech and right-side paralysis. By the time he was brought to a medical center with a stroke acute care unit (the CVA equivalent of the famous coronary care units for heart attacks) he was losing consciousness and was in a coma by nightfall. However, he was fortunate in reaching this specialized facility.

The businessman was cared for by a stroke team, an array of specialists involved directly or on call: internists, neurologists, neurosurgeons, neuropathologists, neuroradiologists (experts in x-rays of the brain), vascular surgeons, psychiatrists, physiatrists (physical medicine experts), specially trained nurses, physical and occupational therapists, plus a host of others with particular interests in CVAs such as ophthalmologists, psychologists, orthopedic surgeons and speech pathologists. The availability of such medical expertise can easily make the difference in whether this seriously ill patient pulls through or not—and this New Yorker did; he was even able to achieve a remarkably complete recovery and to eventually lead a satisfying and active full life.

This businessman was also fortunate in that he suffered his stroke just a couple of years ago and not a couple of decades ago. As Dr. Oscar M. Reinmuth, professor of neurology at the University of Pittsburgh, points out: "As late as the 1950s . . . receiving-room physicians were almost uniformly disinterested in the stroke patient; the flow seemed unending and filled the interns' ward with patients in whom they had no diagnostic interest, for whom they did nothing (on the assumption that there was nothing to be done), and who prevented their admitting 'really interesting cases.' " But this New Yorker's CVA came in a time and situation in which the whole stroke situation had been turned around, for more accurate methods of diagnosis and improved means of treatment and rehabilitation had proved there was hope and help for those with cerebrovascular diseases and so aroused medical interest.

This businessman was fortunate, too, in that his physician saw to it that he received the ultimate in hospital care, because not too many hospitals even today have stroke teams and specialized units for the intensive care of such victims. Dr. Harold Margulies, special assistant in the office of our Assistant Secretary for Health, points out that "the optimum in definitive care for the more complicated cases of . . . stroke requires highly developed medical facilities . . . During the past fifteen years, many changes have taken place in the treatment of stroke." This improvement in medical care is believed by many to be the reason that stroke death rates have fallen more rapidly than those of any other cardiovascular problem. Since 1972, stroke death rates have been dropping at a rate of 5 percent a year.

Nevertheless, the figures indicate the need for the best possible care available in your area should someone in your family suffer a serious or acute stroke. Statistics show that 40 percent of CVA victims still die within a month of their stroke—and 70 to 80 percent of these, according to NINCDS experts, do so within the crucial first ten days. As these experts put it: "Since the outlook for survival depends heavily on the quality of care during this critical period, the need for better 'acute care' is obvious and urgent."

In fact, it is to NINCDS programs that this New Yorker may well owe his life, for that agency has supported a program of stroke acute-care research units in university medical centers and hospitals. These units are equipped for the monitoring of the victim's vital signs (fever, blood pressure, respiration, and the like) and the levels of his brain function, as well as for the treatment of the acute phases of major strokes. Physically these units resemble in many ways the coronary care units that have proved so successful in managing heart attacks and with which most of us have become familiar either through personal experience or TV.

The vital importance of such good medical care in CVAs has been emphasized in a study of the records of two hundred stroke patients by two Northwestern University neurologists, Drs. Meyer Brown and Myron Glassenberg. They found that those who died within a week of their strokes most often did so from brain damage due to the CVAs. But those who lasted longer most often died from causes unrelated to their actual strokes—such as pneumonia, pulmonary embolism (blood clots on the lung), urinary infection, and the like.

We have already seen the anatomy and pathology of the stroke —how a broken blood vessel can produce a hemorrhagic stroke or a blocked artery the far more common ischemic cerebral infarct. However, when infarction occurs there is a sharp disturbance in all the processes and functioning of the brain. Excessive amounts of fluid begin to seep out of the arterioles and capillaries and accumulate in the tissue spaces around the neurons and cerebral structures. Such an excessive accumulation of fluid in tissues is called edema, and this is a major complication of cerebral infarction.

Actually, cerebral infarcts may continue to enlarge for four or five days after the original incident—embolism or thrombosis or whatever—that produced the stroke. Cerebral infarcts are accompanied by this edema, which can of itself produce more widespread and additional involvements. Thus cerebral edema can impair consciousness, disturb many vital functions of the brain, affect vision —often simply through the actual pressure of the fluid on the cerebral hemispheres, the nerves, the centers and the neurons themselves.

When this cerebral edema subsides—usually in a few days by itself or as the result of medical treatment—the victim may once more be able to perform such automatic acts as coughing or swallowing. He may regain consciousness, and even be able to move his paralyzed limbs voluntarily once more; vision may return and many other damaged functions may be regained. Doctors often seek to relieve some of the cerebral edema with medication and support the patient through this period of acute danger until healing and recovery can begin.

When there are massive cerebral infarctions, the edema may be so extensive that the cerebral hemispheres or the entire brain is shifted in its relationships in the skull. Furthermore, the intracranial pressure exerted by this edematous fluid may by itself diminish the already reduced blood flow and normal tissue fluids. Most deaths during the first week after a massive stroke are due to the extensive cerebral edema and increased intracranial pressure, which can displace the cerebral hemispheres downward to the point where they actually interfere with the functioning of the midbrain and lower brain stem, which control the basic vital functions such as respiration and heart action.

But what of the stroke victim himself who enters the hospital—which are the tests and examinations the doctors use to determine his problems and which is the medical treatment then provided; what, too, is the role of blood clotting and platelets, and what is the name of the miracle drug that now promises to actually prevent half of the strokes that result from TIAs? Lastly, where does stress fit into this picture and which are some ways to deal with it to prevent its damage?

The Diagnostic Examination and the Tools Used

The victim of a stroke will receive a typical medical examination at his home or doctor's office, right at the start. Once the physician is certain that the problem is a stroke he will almost always send the patient to the hospital. If the patient is lucky, this will be one with a stroke unit, whether in his own community or one close enough for ambulance transferral. Consultation with a neurologist for diagnosis and treatment will be the next step, to ensure the best possible care. Should there be a possible hemorrhage or other potentially surgical condition present, a neurosurgeon or vascular surgeon may be called in as well, depending on the problem.

The exact patterns of tests will be determined by the initial tentative diagnosis—whether the stroke is hemorrhagic or due to emboli or thrombi, or of uncertain cause (say, a tumor). This preliminary diagnosis is based both on the first physical examination and, even more perhaps, on the history.

Hemorrhagic CVAs, for example, will usually occur during periods of activity, symptoms will appear suddenly and increase in intensity over the first fifteen minutes or so rather than being full-blown at their outset. There will likely be signs of increased intracranial pressure such as vomiting and lethargy. Cerebral emboli—ischemic cerebral infarcts—usually tend to occur in the active, awake patient and the symptoms emerge relatively suddenly. Cerebral thromboses, on the other hand, usually come on during periods of inactivity when blood pressure may be lower, as during sleep.

Obviously the usual blood tests (for lipids, clotting, and the rest) along with a urine examination and a blood-pressure determination are done. The eyes are examined to see if pupils are fixed and how they react to light or movement. Pinpricks or squeezing the nail bed or twisting a toe or finger reveals loss of sensation or even the degree of alteration of consciousness or coma.

The electroencephalogram, or EEG, is well known to people today, since it's been widely used by those who seek to produce alpha waves in the current fad. Actually the EEG was devised half a century ago by a Bavarian physicist and mathematician, Dr. Hans Berger, who turned to medicine and became director of the psychiatric clinic at Jena, Germany. His home-built electroencephalograph revolutionized medicine and the neurosciences when, in 1929, he reported that he had discovered brain waves with it.

The EEG amplifies the electrical currents produced by the brain

—more than a million times, in fact. Under normal circumstances your brain generates 1/10,000 volt in the form of rhythmic oscillating waves, which Berger simply named from the Greek alphabet in the order in which he discovered them. Alpha waves are generated by your brain at eight to twelve cycles per second, beta at thirteen to twenty-five; theta, four to seven; and delta at one to three per second. In sleep, the brain waves slow down to two to three cycles per second—and a special pattern, delta waves, may arise from an area of localized brain-tissue damage.

One of the most commonly performed tests on stroke patients is the so-called spinal tap, or lumbar puncture. A fine needle is inserted through the space between two vertebra and into the spinal canal in the low back—some cerebrospinal fluid (CSF) can be removed and its pressure measured if desired. Laboratory examination of CSF helps doctors in their diagnosis: blood presence may reveal a hemorrhagic stroke, while other cellular or chemical constituents may tell of infection or supply other diagnostic information. Since complications, albeit rare, can occur from spinal taps, these are done only when specific information is being sought and when the specialist feels that the calculated risk involved is worthwhile.

The atom, too, has been turned to medical use and is of help in stroke. In this technique (called "nuclear medicine"), radioisotopes —radioactive substances—are injected into the bloodstream to be carried throughout the body and brain. These isotopes act like so many radio transmitters, sending off their rays as they pass along in the bloodstream. Special cameras and films are used to form images (not too unlike x-rays) of the parts of the body being studied and provide otherwise unobtainable information on the functioning of many parts of the body.

Normally these isotopes remain in the cerebral blood vessels and cannot cross the blood-brain barrier to enter the neural tissues. Called brain scanning, this may give experts the information they need to tell whether the patient has an arteriovenous malformation, an ischemic cerebral infarct or a brain tumor. This radioisotopic brain scanning has an important role in the diagnosis of suspected cerebrovascular disease because it is nondestructive (no damage is done to tissues) and completely nontoxic. As NINCDS experts emphasize: "Neither serious morbidity nor mortality has ever been reported to have resulted from this procedure."

The same cannot be said for an x-ray procedure called angiography. This utilizes a radiopaque material, a substance which blocks x-rays so that it can outline the blood vessels and other areas where there may be blood—like a part of the brain into which blood has leaked from a broken artery. This radiopaque contrast material (its full name) is injected into one of the two carotid arteries to reach the desired cerebral arteries, and as the material passes through the brain a series of x-rays (about a dozen) are taken very rapidly to show the vessels and reveal any malformations or hemorrhages, or any stenosed or occluded vessels.

But, as these NINCDS experts point out: "All forms of angiography still entail a calculated risk to the patient." For this reason and for one other, angiography is only now used under special circumstances when the calculated risk has to be taken. The reason for this is that angiography has been known to cause seizures and neurological deficits such as blindness or even partial or complete paralysis of one or more extremities. While these deficits usually are transient, they can be permanent.

The other reason for the near-abandonment of angiography is the Nobel Prize-winning development of what experts term computed tomography, or CT scan. This highly sophisticated x-ray machine and technique introduced in 1972 produces marvelously precise pictures of the human body. A pencil-thin beam of x-rays is directed with pinpoint accuracy and rotated about the body part to produce images of layers of brain or other tissue, each about one centimeter (less than a half-inch) thick. These images are then processed by computers to produce three-dimensional pictures a hundred times more sensitive than conventional x-rays are to changes in these tissues. It has since been amply demonstrated, according to Dr. Thomas P. Naidich, professor of radiology at Washington University Medical School, that CT is superior to all other diagnostic tests in detection and localization of brain lesions as well as in the accuracy and specificity of diagnosis.

Dr. Naidich finds it the first choice for suspected cerebral hemorrhage and believes every suspected stroke victim should undergo a CT scan. Moreover, this scan is as simple and innocuous as a head x-ray. At Massachusetts General Hospital it has been found that with CT scanning available, angiograms were canceled for twenty-five of thirty-six patients during one short period alone. Not surprisingly, the 1979 Nobel Prize for Physiology or Medicine went to the developers of CT: an English electronics engineer, Godfrey Newbold Hounsfield, and an American Tufts University professor of physics, Allan MacLeod Cormack. Working entirely independently and unaware of each other, the two pioneered this development.

Ophthalmodynamometry (ODM) is a simple, harmless and repeatable test which can detect three quarters of unilateral carotid stenosis. By applying either pressure or suction to the eye and watching its inside blood vessels with an ophthalmoscope (the device used to inspect the inside of your eyes), systolic and diastolic readings can be taken, and if the eyes differ by 20 percent, a carotid artery obstruction—stenosis, plaques, thrombi—is likely to be present.

There are a variety of other, less used tests. There is thermography: skin temperature varies in relation to the blood flow and this is a simple test to measure the infrared or heat emissions from the body surface. It identifies 85 percent of those in whom there is a marked stenosis or occlusion of one of the carotid arteries.

Ultrasonography, or echoencephalography, is another useful technique. This uses short (two hundred to two thousand times a second) pulses of ultrasound (sound at too high a level to be heard by the human ear, "silent sound"). The sound signal is directed at body structures: tissues with differing densities will reflect the sound signal differently so that it can be recorded on an oscilloscope (like your TV screen) or turned into a picture. The accuracy of such tests is roughly 90 percent that of x-rays. It is particularly useful for brain studies, since it produces no radiation or discomfort, and shifts of midline structures in the brain can be seen in cerebral infarction, hemorrhage, edema and other brain disorders. New means of diagnosis continue to be introduced and hopefully will continue to improve the diagnosis and location of cerebral problems as well as providing better means than ever before of evaluating and determining . . .

The Medical Treatment of Stroke

Treatment of stroke has four basic aims: to save the life of the victim; to limit, as far as possible, the amount of brain damage; to reduce the person's disability and disfigurement; and, finally, to prevent another stroke. These ends are sought in just about this order. The need for expert medical care is very apparent, for there are sometimes two possible approaches—the medical (treatment by medication) and the surgical (treatment by operation or manipulation)—and a decision between them must be made. When such a determination is to be reached, the specialist in cerebrovascular disorders is needed.

Almost invariably today, the stroke victim is hospitalized—and if possible in an institution with a stroke center or unit, or at least an intensive-care unit. After a careful physical examination in which blood pressure is checked, drugs may be used to ensure that any hypertension is brought under control, although often diastolic pressures of 100 or 110 are thought acceptable in the completed-stroke victim, but this is a highly individual medical decision.

Respiration is an absolute essential to life and is one of the first considerations in the medical care of the stroke victim, particularly a comatose one. It may be necessary to insert breathing tubes through nose or mouth, or even a tracheostomy (an incision in the neck to give direct access by tubes in the windpipe whereby air can reach the lungs unhindered) may be needed. Oxygen is often administered to CVA victims. And routinely, in stroke or intensive-care units, the patient's heart is continuously monitored by an electrocardiograph, so the family need not be alarmed when they find that an electrocardiogram (EKG) has been taken—these various measures are for the protection of the victim and not necessarily because the medical situation is excessively grave. In fact, the use of oxygen and the EKG should be regarded as assurances that proper care is available and being provided to the stroke victim.

Blood pressure is one of the first concerns. Mayo Clinic studies have shown hypertension to be present in 62 to 89 percent of those with cerebral hemorrhage, and we have already seen how common it is in those with nonhemorrhagic strokes. Throughout the care of the acute phase of CVA, patients in stroke or intensive-care units, the arterial blood pressure is checked and recorded at least every hour.

Naturally, the neurological status—the victim's responses to various special tests—is observed very carefully. A "watch sheet" (a standard evaluation form) makes it possible to specifically report the changes so that these can be interpreted uniformly by all those concerned with the medical care of the patient.

In the acute phases of a stroke, the victim is cared for in bed with his head slightly raised. Should he be having difficulties with vomiting or oral or nasal secretions which put him in danger of inhaling this material, he may be placed on his side or stomach (even with his head down so that gravity helps prevent inhalation of such material). Raising the head also lowers the cerebral venous pressure and may reduce cerebral congestion and edema.

Body temperature, too, is watched closely because its elevation can mean either infection or a severe disturbance of the vital centers affecting temperature control. Infection calls for prompt diagnosis, and when the cause is bacterial, the use of antibiotics to bring this promptly under control. Hypothermia (lowered body temperature) can slow the cerebral metabolism, reduce the amount of oxygen and nutrients needed, protect the brain from reduced blood supply and combat edema. Temperature is lowered by positioning the patient between a pair of thermal blankets or even using bags of ice if more rapid reduction is desired. NINCDS experts point out that limited experience with hypothermia has left its role and value in stroke treatment still uncertain.

In comatose stroke patients, intravenous fluids and feeding is used for the first few days. A nasal tube extending into the stomach (the so-called nasogastric tube) is inserted; after three days this tube may be used for feeding the patient. Urinary output is watched closely during this period, and a catheter may have to be inserted.

Physicians have a considerable number of drugs they use for

treating the victims of ischemic cerebral infarction. These agents fall into four classes, each of which is used for a different purpose in the attempt to deal with the various aspects of the stroke.

The vasodilators are intended to do what their name says—to dilate the blood vessels, and in this way, to compensate for the reduced blood supply which produced the stroke. The most potent of these drugs is carbon dioxide. A mixture of 5 percent carbon dioxide and 95 percent oxygen has been used widely in acute strokes, but experts today question the real effectiveness of such therapy (for there are a number of drugs available for this purpose). Some evidence indicates that these drugs may in fact reduce the amount of blood to ischemic areas by shunting it away to the normal brain tissue or lowering the general systemic (body) blood pressure.

The vasodepressors and vasopressors are the blood-pressure-lowering drugs and are widely used in strokes, since so many CVAs are preceded by long-standing hypertension. A large number of these drugs are used today and sometimes, in urgent situations, even intravenously at six-hour intervals (with careful monitoring to avoid the opposite problem of low blood pressure). Other drugs may be given intramuscularly or by mouth if the patient can take it this way (obviously the comatose can not). These are usually given at frequent intervals in smaller doses because a single large one usually fails to bring hypertension down. Too rapid a drop in tension is always avoided and sometimes doctors prefer to keep arterial pressure somewhat above normal to ensure an adequate cerebral blood flow to the damaged brain.

The anticoagulants—drugs which prevent the blood from clotting, or coagulating—are used by experts in the progressing or evolving strokes. Here, however, doctors make sure that the stroke is the ischemic or nonhemorrhagic kind and use regular blood tests to be certain that the ability to clot remains within safe limits. Such patients are carefully watched to be certain there is no bleeding elsewhere in the body nor any signs of intracranial bleeding.

The most commonly used of these anticoagulants is heparin, a natural body product which normally acts as a safeguard to prevent your blood from clotting by itself in your body and its blood vessels. Heparin must be given intravenously and in the stroke patient is commonly given by continuous infusion into a vein. For the long term, doctors use warfarin, a so-called coumarin anticoagulant, which can be taken by mouth. However, a large number of other drugs will interact with warfarin so that, for example, aspirin, oral contraceptives, phenobarbital, some antibiotics and many other medications must be carefully avoided. Anyone on these so-called blood thinners should check carefully with his doctor before also taking any over-the-counter or old prescription medicines.

The uncontrolled increase in intracranial pressure produced by cerebral edema is one of the most common causes of death from stroke. Ideally, doctors would be able to control this edema effectively and uniformly over as much time as is needed for the brain's self-recovery and self-healing to take place, but as yet there is neither drug nor method to attain this end.

Dehydrating agents have been used for the past half-century, starting with concentrated solutions of dextrose (grape or corn sugar) given intravenously to reduce this edema. Corticosteroids (hormones of the adrenal gland such as cortisone) have been widely used for this purpose, and while effective in those with brain tumors, are of uncertain value in stroke victims. Urea and glycerol solutions, too, have been used. A solution of mannitol (an alcohol derived from fruit sugar and used as the basis of dietary sweets) given intravenously can produce a drop in intracranial pressure within a few minutes and has its maximal effect within a half-hour to an hour: this has proved valuable in life-threatening situations or when time is needed in which to prepare for surgery.

Obviously the best hope in stroke will always be prevention and that is actually possible today, as we will now see.

Your Blood and How It Clots

This really is the world of thrombi and of emboli. Nature has had to achieve a sort of juggling effect in man's bloodstream. Without an ability to clot, the slightest tear or injury to a blood vessel would cause us to bleed to death—but if the blood clotted in our arteries or veins, we could not survive, either. Actually a complex two-part system has been devised, so there are two different types of drugs which are needed to deal with the stroke problems and, it is hoped, to prevent them as well.

Each cubic millimeter of blood contains a quarter to a half million disc-shaped specks about 1/25,000 inch each—the blood platelets. These platelets contain a number of chemical compounds, including cephalin, which activates an enzyme that acts on a blood protein to produce fibrin, an insoluble, stringy, tough gel.

When a blood vessel is injured—whether it's torn or even when the intima is injured—the blood platelets somehow become sticky and adhere to the injured surface and to each other. When there is a hole or cut end of a vessel, the platelets initially stick together to form a plug that seals the mouth of the bleeding vessel and stops the hemorrhage. Once the bleeding has been stopped by the platelet plug, a network of fibrin is formed by the action on the blood initiated by the chemicals in the platelets so that a tough composite seal is formed. This seal can withstand the full force of the arterial blood pressure and prevent bleeding until permanent healing has taken place.

Were the platelets deficient or chemically altered, the initial bleeding would not stop. On the other hand, were something to block the process leading to the formation of fibrin and to the final tough clot, the friable platelet plug would soon be swept away and a delayed bleeding would start at some later time—these are known as disorders of coagulation and happen in hemophiliacs.

Two kinds of drugs can affect normal clotting: anticoagulating agents (those interfering with fibrin formation) and platelet antiagglutinating agents (those preventing platelets from sticking together). So theoretically one should be able to prevent strokes in the victims of TIAs, since these most commonly occur from atherosclerosis with platelet accumulations, and clots on vessel walls breaking off to form emboli. And it would seem one might be able to do this with agents that can perform either one of these two actions to prevent clotting.

The use of anticoagulants—such as warfarin or heparin—has

been shown in some studies to sharply reduce the strokes that result from TIAs. However, some of the results appear doubtful. There are suggestions that this approach works better for those with emboli—and some reports question whether anticoagulants either increase survival or reduce the incidence of resultant strokes. In fact, an NINCDS team of national experts concludes: "The risk of serious hemorrhage from protracted use of oral anticoagulants outweighs many potential advantages."

The great danger of such therapy is hemorrhage anywhere in the body; another disadvantage is that such patients must be carefully monitored with regular and frequent blood tests to keep the coagulating level of the blood within safe limits.

But now it has been proved scientifically and conclusively that we can cut strokes in half—with a safe, well-known, easily obtainable and inexpensive drug that needs no monitoring and little supervision once started, and that affects not the coagulation but the platelets themselves.

The New Miracle Drug for Stroke Prevention!

Fifteen years ago Dr. Harvey J. Weiss, director of hematology at New York City's Roosevelt Hospital, performed a series of classical scientific studies on a chemical called acetylsalicylic acid. Actually, this is the world's most widely used drug (Americans alone take fifty billion tablets of it and its compounds annually), and you know it as aspirin. When Dr. Weiss began his studies there were bits and pieces of evidence indicating that aspirin could prevent heart attack and stroke by interfering with clotting, but there was no scientifically acceptable proof.

This hematologist deliberately injured the intima of neck and thigh arteries in dogs to some of whom he was giving aspirin. Not a single vessel was completely blocked by a blood clot among those on aspirin, while virtually half the arteries in the untreated dogs suffered this fate. Dr. Weiss found that the bleeding time (how long it takes for blood to stop flowing from a forearm puncture) remained prolonged for as much as a week by a single dose of aspirin.

"Aspirin irreversibly damages the entire population of platelets present in the body throughout their entire life," he explains. In short, one aspirin tablet can affect all the blood platelets in the body until they are replaced (as they normally are) every week to ten days. It's clear too that it is the acetyl part of aspirin that does this, because sodium salicylate won't do it. This so-called acetylation of the platelets somehow keeps them from sticking to each other. One theory is that somehow the acetyl radical becomes bound to the platelet cell membrane and keeps it from rupturing and sticking when it touches the wall of the damaged artery.

With this and other scattered pieces of evidence, two major, carefully conceived and scientifically valid, definitive studies were begun. Their final conclusive proof came in 1978 in Canada and in Houston, Texas. The Canadian study involved some six hundred patients scattered across the country from the fishing fleets of Newfoundland to the logging camps of Vancouver Island, and in twelve university centers. This research continued from the fall of 1971 until the summer of 1977. All the subjects had suffered TIAs and followed a regimen of four aspirin tablets a day—to achieve an amazing but male chauvinist success. The leader of this Canadian trial, Dr. J. M. Barnett, University Hospital, London, Ontario, summarizes their findings: ". . . there was a reduction of stroke and death approaching 50 percent among men." But why women failed to benefit he admits "remains to be explained; hormonal factors may be involved."

On the heels of this study Dr. William S. Fields, professor of neurology at Houston's University of Texas, reported his own scientifically acceptable study of over three hundred patients. Starting in 1973, he also found a statistically significant lower incidence of major strokes when he gave two aspirin twice a day to his subjects. As he points out, the Canadian study and his own both confirm the exciting fact that "aspirin reduces or results in cessation of TIAs and that among males there is a 50 percent reduction in death and disability from stroke."

So persuasive and conclusive has this evidence proved that neurologists and other physicians (for example, a professor of neurology in New York and another in Detroit, an East Coast internist) are commonly prescribing four aspirin a day for patients threatened with stroke. And there is some thought that even fewer aspirin may actually be necessary than the currently accepted four-a-day regime, which is purely arbitrary anyhow.

Dr. John S. Meyer, a professor of neurology at Houston's Baylor College of Medicine and also involved in similar research, sums up the situation today: "Aspirin appears to be very helpful in patients at risk for major strokes. It can be used early on in the disease process when vigorous treatment is important. It also seems to reverse the disease process among patients who have had a major stroke. Aspirin is the drug of choice, as well as the less expensive medication."

The precise role and dosage of aspirin is something to be determined in the future, but it must be remembered that this drug—for all its seeming safety—can be dangerous to some people. About two persons in every thousand are allergic to it, and for them it can even be fatal. Others have to take it in special ways to avoid damage from it. Aspirin must be kept from children; it is the chief cause of accidental death among them. Adults taking varied medications or with certain health problems should not use aspirin—for example, those using anticoagulants or gout medication, those with stomach ulcers or hearing problems, and so on. In short, people taking any regular medication or those with allergies (asthma in particular) or any chronic health problems should check with their doctor before using aspirin, for it can be a double-edged sword and do more harm than good.

Stress and Stroke

Stress is always with you. Whether you run to catch a bus or deal with unpleasantness on your job or have a fight with your family, the manifestations of stress are always the same: your heart pounds and you breathe hard, your blood pressure rises and your pupils dilate, your palms get sweaty and your stomach ties in knots, your digestion grinds to a halt.

Stress is essential, however, for it prepares you to put out to the maximum as sugar is poured into your blood to provide instantly available fuel for quick energy. The heavy breathing provides more oxygen and gets rid of the extra carbon dioxide of intense activity. Red blood cells flood the bloodstream to carry more oxygen to active muscles and brain, to take away carbon dioxide. Blood-clotting mechanisms are enhanced so that too much blood won't be lost in the event of an injury. The heart speeds up and the blood pressure rises so that fuel and oxygen are always available and the waste products eliminated. Muscles are prepared for greater efforts. Extra adrenaline brings the body to peak functioning, and digestion is shut down so its blood supply is free to be sent where it's most needed, to muscles and brain.

But stress also puts a strain on your body—and if there is any weakness, it may push your body over the edge. If, for example, you already have hypertension, the new rise may be too much for already weakened arteries to cope with the added pressure. While its role in stroke has never been absolutely proved—that you can "have a stroke" if you get too excited or live too stressful a life—there is a lot of evidence pointing in that direction.

Back in September 1974, Dr. Samuel Silverman, a Harvard professor of psychiatry, told *Time* magazine that President Richard Nixon's areas of greatest psychosomatic susceptibility were his legs and lungs. Based on Nixon's known medical records and a psychological assessment, Dr. Silverman pointed to the likelihood of a thrombus from his leg phlebitis (vein inflammation) producing an embolus to lodge in his lungs. When this actually happened only a few days later, the psychiatrist became virtually a folk hero, a prophet in his own right. Many other physicians were also convinced that these thrombi and emboli were related to the stress of the Watergate scandal and his forced resignation in an atmosphere of public condemnation.

In a study of air traffic controllers (high-stress work) and of second-class airmen (relatively stress-free tasks), investigators found that hypertension, peptic ulcer and diabetes occurred several times more often in the high-stress jobholders than in men in the relatively stress-free occupation.

Experts advise a variety of ways to bring stress down to bearable levels—if you want to stay healthy. If the work you do is too much for you, too tension-producing, it may be well worth your life to seek another and less stress-filled job. Blow off steam in recreation: play a hard game of squash or tennis, see a funny movie or show, listen to music you enjoy, take a vacation away from it all. As a matter of fact, learning to take things philosophically is one of the best and oldest known ways of relaxing.

But if these things don't help, a talk with your doctor may be of value—or some more specialized professional help may well be in order. Psychotherapy may solve problems that nothing else can, but somehow we all should learn to keep stress at a level we can be comfortable with—and which will not harm us. Millions are striving for this through a variety of methods ranging from yoga to transcendental meditation and including a whole host of methods. But stress must be kept at a bearable level—for nothing is ever worth the price of a stroke.

9

THE SURGICAL ATTACK ON STROKE

Prevention, Relief and Cure under the Microscope

The man in his mid-sixties came into his local hospital complaining of difficulty in speech and weakness in his right hand. The hospital —only thirty or fourty miles from Boston—called Dr. Robert M. Crowell at Boston's famous Massachusetts General Hospital (MGH). An ambulance picked up the man promptly but by the time it reached MGH the man was already suffering a major stroke, with his speech completely gone, the right side of his body totally paralyzed.

MGH has its own stroke center, so it was fully prepared to deal with this emergency. An angiogram revealed a blockage in the carotid artery and Dr. Crowell, a Harvard and MGH professor of surgery, tells the story: "At surgery we were able to remove this blockage and restore a normal blood flow. Almost immediately, in the recovery room, the patient to some degree was able to move and speak. He has since gone on to make a 95 percent recovery." As the neurosurgeon sums this up: "We caught him in time. If he had not been treated as promptly as he was, I'm sure he would be institutionalized today."

This is just one story of the amazing accomplishments of surgery for stroke today. True, it's not all one way—but this story does emphasize again the importance of the stroke center with its ever-ready status, its vast specialized staff and its high level of every kind of needed medical expertise. This also shows the payoff—and the importance of seeing to it that anyone suffering an attack gets, if possible, to a properly equipped stroke center. Surgery can be lifesaving but there are those who urge rethinking the use of some stroke surgery should it be advised. These experts implore you to ask questions beforehand because under certain circumstances and in some institutions this surgery can carry a complication and mortality rate five times as high as it should be. To protect yourself and your family, you should know the story of both stroke and stroke-prevention surgery.

The New World of Microsurgery

Brain surgery, a part of neurosurgery, is very new and, in a real sense too, very old—for it is both a Stone Age technique and a Space Age skill. Some medical historians even believe that brain surgery was actually the first form of surgery that man practiced and that it came long before any other. For headache sufferers and victims of epilepsy, perhaps for the insane as well (to allow demons to escape from the head), Stone Age medicine men would perform an operation called trephining, the cutting out of circular pieces of bone from the skull.

Operating on living subjects (patients, if you will), these Stone Age practitioners sometimes removed as many as five pieces of bone from a single skull. By the Neolithic period this was actually a widespread practice. The surgery was performed with primitive but highly effective surgical instruments made of stone—some were, in fact, merely flint knives. The holes achieved in this way varied in size up to several inches in diameter and sometimes comprised a goodly part of the skull.

This is a delicate operation even today and often carries a high rate of mortality with it. These ancient medical practitioners no doubt performed this surgery without anesthesia and with no knowledge of anatomy, physiology or infection. The astounding thing is that modern scientific examinations of these ancient tre-phined skulls has shown that many of these subjects survived at least for years after their surgery, as evidenced by the fact that new bone had time to grow around the edges of the holes thus created in their skulls.

This was apparently a universal Stone Age practice, for trephined skulls have turned up all over the world except in Australia and some parts of the Far East and Africa. Much of our understanding of how this was done with primitive tools comes from some actual observations made in this century of similar practices, particularly in the Aures Mountains in Algeria, because trephining is still being performed in many other parts of the world, including Melanesia and the Caucasus.

Modern neurosurgery began a hundred years ago, in the early 1880s, when Sir William Macewen, professor of surgery at the University of Glasgow, was one of the first to drain a brain abscess. He reported an astonishing success with twenty-three of twenty-four of his early patients—at a time when the mortality rate approached 100 percent with this operation; it still carries a tragically high 40 percent mortality rate (although today the less serious ones can be cured without surgery thanks to antibiotics).

From Macewen's time until the early twentieth century, surgeons suddenly turned, in considerable numbers, to brain surgery for tumors—only to find half their patients dying on the operating table, and the successes very rare. Even the few competent neurosurgeons had mortality rates of 30 to 80 percent. The close of the last century saw the development of a technique which opened the way to successful brain surgery and whose use makes possible the latest surgical assault on stroke.

To reach the brain it was then necessary to drill a hole in the skull and then enlarge it with chisels. This was crude and left much to be desired, and cutting out a circular plate of bone with hammer and chisel was also excessively traumatic. An Italian gynecologist, Leonardo Gigli, devised the modern technique of drilling several holes in a semicircle and then connecting them with a flexible saw passed through one hole and out the next so that the flap of bone could be lifted out—a technique termed a "craniotomy"—although electric saws are now also being used.

But it was the great Harvey Cushing, first at Johns Hopkins and then at Harvard, who turned neurosurgery into a true specialty and proved what could be accomplished. Starting about 1905, Cushing began his amazing advances by devising and developing the use of tiny clips of silver wire which he handled with special forceps to "clip" or compress the cerebral blood vessels and thus control the surgical hemorrhaging that then was the bane of neurosurgeons. He simply left the clips in place after his operation was completed. In fact, his techniques are now being used in the struggle against hemorrhagic strokes where neurosurgeons must enter the brain to tie off or clip the defective vessels to stop the bleeding.

Cushing dramatically proved how delicacy of touch and new techniques could improve on the mortality rates from brain surgery achieved by the leading surgeons of his day. Where the best averages ranged roughly from 50 to 75 percent, depending on the operation, Cushing had, by 1927, brought his own mortality rates down to a startlingly low 4 percent. His rates, in fact, compare very favorably with those of today with all our advances in anesthesia, antibiotics and sophisticated equipment.

The new technique which has made it possible for the first time for surgeons to perform operations never before thought possible is microsurgery. It has opened the way to prevent strokes and their recurrences, even to help the neurological deficits or losses occasioned by previous strokes. It is microsurgery, in fact, that has made possible such surgery as Dr. Crowell succeeded with at MGH.

During a typical operation two doctors, masked and gowned, sit peering intently through binocular microscope eyepieces set on opposite sides of a device which, suspended from above, could almost pass for a submarine periscope. Their hands barely moving under the microscope, they concentrate on the figure stretched out on the table between them. There is almost no sound in the room except for the words and curt orders passing between surgeon and assistant and other similarly garbed figures moving quietly and efficiently about. A miniature camera, movie or TV, records what is going on under the microscope through a third eyepiece set off to the side between the doctors. Everything is as sterile and controlled as human ingenuity can make it.

In the little more than quarter century since microsurgery first made its appearance, this new discipline has been developed to an amazing degree of sophistication in both technique and equipment, along with a broad and growing range of applications. From its use in ear surgery, where it was first utilized, it spread to eye surgery and then to neurosurgery, to hand and plastic surgery. It has become established as an essential surgical technique and is practiced in every advanced country in the world today.

Repeatedly, neurosurgeons emphasize to me that the future of neurosurgery lies in microsurgery, which has already opened a whole new era here. One well-known neurosurgeon said frankly about certain nerve tumors: "If I didn't have an operating microscope, I either wouldn't operate or I'd send the patient to a surgeon who did have one."

By enlarging the operating field some ten to forty times, the faintest quiver of a microsurgeon's hands becomes so magnified that it looks like the wave of a giant's paw. In fact, many microsurgeons will not even have a cup of coffee the night before they operate because the caffeine may cause sufficient tremor to be markedly noticeable under such enlargements. Nerves and blood vessels invisible to the naked eye suddenly look as big as the thumb on your hand. The usual very definite movements of a surgeon's hands must be converted to very subtle and carefully controlled and virtually exquisite movements. Pneumatic devices, even, are now used because under many circumstances the human hand, no matter how steady and supported, cannot always adequately control the miniaturized materials and instruments, some almost invisible to the naked eye.

These operating microscopes have zoom lenses, and pedals so that their lenses can be moved, changed, focused and controlled by the surgeon's foot, for he cannot take his hands away from the surgical field. Unique specialized instruments have been developed —scissors with blades 1/16 inch long and a shaft the thickness of a match stick, whose blades operate by compressed air instead of opening and closing on a hinge. It's possible with such techniques to put fifty-eight stitches along a three-quarter-inch incision in an artery 1/10 inch in diameter—and to use thread one-fourth the thickness of a human hair and needles the thickness of two red blood cells, roughly 1/5,000 inch in diameter.

But what of the surgeons who operate in this strange miniature but vital world? Dr. Horst Wullstein, one of the great international pioneers in ear surgery and professor at Germany's University of Würzburg, explained to me: "I am the son of a surgeon and know the development of surgery since the beginning of this century, even at home as a boy. Surgeons with those wonderful hands always existed, but they are rare. Microsurgery forces the surgeon to become much more delicate and I feel we are getting a new type of surgeon—the rough general surgeon will slowly disappear."

According to Professor Wullstein, the microsurgeon's mind must switch gears in order to change from the rough, large movements of ordinary surgery to the precise, delicate motions needed under the microscope: "If you are the right man for this kind of work, you have a sense of space and depth. If you can really see and know what you intend to do, your hand will obey. This shifting to another dimension within yourself is what's so very tiring—holding your arms so very very quiet costs you strength and particularly causes mental fatigue."

As the microsurgery pioneer points out, Zeiss developed a real operating microscope only after World War II and introduced it for the first time at the International Congress of Otolaryngology (ear, nose and throat specialty) in Amsterdam in 1953. As he recalls: "I got their second or third microscope and started in 1953 with this. But otological [ear] surgery without the microscope is no more possible. By 1960 Zeiss told me they had sold two thousand or more operating microscopes in otology but none in the other specialties. No young otologists can be properly trained today without being trained in microsurgery—it is the new dimension in surgery."

NINCDS experts describe the change microsurgery has produced in stroke thus: "In the past, cerebrovascular surgery has been limited almost entirely to correction of flaws or blockages . . . in the larger arteries such as the carotid arteries . . . In recent years, intracranial arteries have come within reach of the surgeon. With the operating microscope, it is possible to remove clots from very small vessels, and also to make grafts [transplants] of very small blood vessels down to one millimeter [1/25 inch] in diameter." These experts even point to a four-week-old infant who was operated on for hemorrhagic stroke from a tiny middle cerebral artery aneurysm (a bulging weak spot in the vessel wall). Since there were severe neurological deficits from this hemorrhage, an operation was indicated—and eventually the infant had a complete return of function.

Emergency or Preventive Surgery

A stroke is an emergency in which prompt action alone can save lives. Surgeons are now urging that such action can also prevent disability and reduce the effects of stroke as well. In stroke—as in heart attacks—the speed with which the victims are sent to the proper hospital emergency room can make a big difference in the final outcome of these major health crises.

Dr. Robert Crowell warns the medical profession and the public alike: "There's too much pessimism about stroke among the public and physicians in general." And he adds: "As a result, too many people languish for hours or even days in the process of having a stroke because no one realizes that they can intervene and make a difference. In many instances the stroke takes hours, not minutes."

What the MGH neurosurgeon looks to for help is the operation we mentioned at the very beginning of this chapter—the so-called carotid endarterectomy. Before we go into the evidence and successes which both Dr. Crowell and others have produced to show there may be a new way to prevent the damage even when a stroke has already begun, let us look at the operation of which they speak and the condition underlying it.

The patients are essentially victims of carotid atherosclerosis in which the affected vessel becomes increasingly stenosed or occluded by the plaque. This condition continues until either a stroke in evolution (as happened to the Massachusetts man we mentioned earlier) occurs or the victim's TIAs worsen so steadily that a full-fledged stroke looms close ahead. A number of neurosurgeons and vascular surgeons are now performing emergency operations on these patients to restore the blood flow to the starved brain before it is permanently damaged and an infarct results.

The surgery itself is—as compared with many other neurosurgical procedures—relatively simple. First, however, there is need for emergency angiography to locate the blockage and reveal both its extent, the length of artery involved, and the degree of stenosis (95 percent reduction in the lumen of the artery in TIAs was considered by some to be necessary grounds for such emergency surgery).

The carotids are quite easy to reach through an incision in the neck made near where the plaque is located. Surgeons commonly use a shunt, or bypass, to maintain and even increase blood supply to the brain during surgery. A large-bore needle, pointed toward the chest, is inserted below the level of the proposed surgery, while another pointed toward the head is inserted above this level. The two needles are connected by a tube so that the blood can be detoured around the occluded section, and the brain supplied with blood. However, if the blood flow in the opposite carotid and through the circle of Willis is judged adequate to nourish the brain sufficiently during surgery, a shunt is not used.

The section of artery to be operated on is now clamped shut both above and below the blockage, and the artery slit open to expose its inside. The atheromatous plaque is scooped out as one might a papaya or melon, leaving the rind or skin—in this case the wall of the artery—untouched. The artery is now carefully sewed shut and microsurgery helps to make sure that this is done properly so that there will be no leakage. When clamps and bypass are removed, the reamed-out section of the artery fills with blood and starts to pulsate as it should while the brain once more obtains its proper blood supply.

Carotid endarterectomy has in the past been considered dangerous in acute strokes due to the fear that cerebral hemorrhages would result in damaged areas of the brain following surgery. Dr. Crowell disagrees, for he feels such patients can now be adequately protected after surgery by careful control of their blood pressure. However, NINCDS experts point to some studies which have shown that mortality rates in patients with acute strokes are twice as great among those treated surgically as among those treated medically—and when surgery was postponed for two weeks or more, the surgical mortality was greatly reduced.

Some new evidence may eventually turn this whole picture around. The MGH neurosurgeon now has shown the results of this emergency carotid endarterectomy in fifty-five patients brought to the MGH emergency room while suffering from moderate or severe stroke. These were people who had neurological deficits such as one-sided weakness or impaired speech. They were promptly given angiography, and if an obstruction of the carotid was found, immediately moved to the operating room. Some were taken to the operating room within two hours, and all underwent surgery within twenty-four hours.

Of the fifty-five patients, thirty-six were diagnosed as mild to moderate strokes, and the results obtained with these Dr. Crowell terms "encouraging," for he has had a good to excellent progress in 80 percent and only one death. However, the results in those with massive strokes were poor, for seven of the nineteen in whom this emergency operation was attempted died. The surgeon admits that there seems no likelihood the operation will help such patients, and he has therefore abandoned the procedure for these.

Other surgeons are also taking a new look at emergency carotid endarterectomies. Dr. Jerry Goldstone, a University of California/ San Francisco professor of surgery, and Dr. Wesley S. Moore, University of Arizona professor of surgery, have performed these operations on twenty-six patients with either mild or moderate stroke-in-evolution or TIAs which were building up in severity— but none with severe strokes. Every one of those operated on made a complete neurological recovery following the procedure.

Only a few major medical centers are doing this operation on an emergency basis. Dr. Crowell frankly sums up its current status: "We have highly suggestive evidence that the operation helps in many cases, although it is *not* proven beyond a doubt. A number of people can't be helped and the results differ among hospitals." He points out, too, that people vary greatly in their resistance to stroke just as they do in their recovery from it.

In short, here is an exciting but still experimental new hope which only the future can prove out or discard as experience with it increases. And Dr. Crowell warns honestly: "This is not miracle surgery. But in our hands, most patients improved to 'good' status; they were able to function as they did before, or at least were independent." Its success, as he emphasizes, depends on a team approach of the hospital staff—and above all else, on early detection of stroke.

This MGH surgeon would like to see more public awareness of this hope and the problem, with more widespread understanding: "One problem is that the patient shows up several hours after the stroke begins. . . . My dream is that alert family members will recognize the condition immediately and get help. Then drug treatment might be started and the patient can be evaluated for surgery, if appropriate."

Sometimes trauma can produce a stroke and emergency carotid endarterectomy may produce dramatic results here too. One middle-aged man was punched on the right side of his neck and became unconscious five minutes later. He came to in about an hour to find his left side partially paralyzed and his tongue weak. Emergency endarterectomy was performed and a thrombus found and removed. Five days later neurologic recovery began and by a month after his surgery, 90 percent of his function had been restored. Occlusion of the carotid can occur in children following trauma to the neck area, and surgery is often utilized on an emergency basis.

What You Should Know About the Dangers of Carotid Surgery

It is now more than a quarter century since an English surgeon reported the successful treatment by carotid endarterectomy of a sixty-six-year-old woman who during a five-month period suffered thirty-three TIAs, resulting in slurred speech, numbness and weakness of her right arm and leg. Yet the picture still remains unclear and confused—which patients should be operated on and when, what conditions are best dealt with surgically and at what stage, even how safe the operation itself is.

Dr. Jack P. Whisnant, Mayo Clinic professor of neurology, and his colleagues find that "the value of surgical treatment in the prevention of stroke remains unproven." And a NINCDS study group headed by Dr. James Toole agrees: "The question of whether to operate on patients with occlusion of an internal carotid artery is controversial." They point out, however, that this operation has been considered of value in preventing strokes when the victim of the TIAs also has angiographic proof of severe stenosis in the carotid artery involved.

Most surgeons will not recommend this operation unless there is at least a 70 percent reduction in the diameter of the lumen of the involved artery or an ulcerated atherosclerotic plaque. (When these plaques become ulcerated they are especially likely to cause emboli because pieces of thrombi break off these ulcers, for some still unclear reason.)

Carotid endarterectomy is the most widely practiced operation to prevent strokes. An estimated hundred thousand such procedures are performed annually in the United States, so you should be aware of the warnings experts issue. NINCDS experts say that "carotid surgical procedures must be carried out in a facility where the operative team is experienced in surgery on small arteries, familiar with surgical hazards, and capable of managing any ensuing complications."

One of our leading experts on stroke also has a warning very specifically for the public. Dr. William K. Hass, New York University professor of neurology and chairman of the American Heart Association [AHA] Council on Stroke, advises that before anyone goes ahead with a carotid endarterectomy he should ask his surgeon two questions:

1. How many of these do you do? and
2. How well do you do? [in short, the mortality and morbidity rates he has achieved with this operation]

Despite the large numbers performed there is a wide variation in experience, for active surgical teams do as many as thirty a month while some community-hospital surgeons may do only three a year. While there can be setbacks in the course of any surgery, the complication rates for this endarterectomy even in large community hospitals can be as much as five times too high.

As Dr. Hass emphasizes: "Our message is that surgical treatment of the warning signs of stroke [TIAs] . . . should be based on a medical-surgical judgment which must as its first consideration take into account the quality of the surgical team, their batting average."

Experts like Dr. Hass had their attention first called to this problem by a 1977 report in the highly respected AHA journal *Stroke*. A series of more than two hundred carotid endarterectomies performed by eleven qualified neurological and vascular surgeons in two community hospitals were studied. Among those patients with TIAs, 18 percent suffered strokes, exactly what the operation was intended to prevent.

Comparing these results with several hundred similar procedures at major medical-school teaching hospitals, the New York neurologist found the average complication rate to be under 5 percent. However, he regards even this as excessively higher than the "acceptable" rate of 3 percent. Another study has shown that some surgical teams report less than 2 percent complication rates.

The Mayo team also feels that the skill of the surgeon should be a factor in determining whether TIA patients would undergo surgery. As this team points out, morbidity and mortality rates for these endarterectomies have been brought down to what they consider acceptable levels—less than 2 percent—in some centers while in some community hospitals these rates may go as high as 21 percent.

On the other hand, a 1979 study of more than a hundred endarterectomies performed in a North Dakota community hospital reveals mortality and morbidity rates of 1 percent. So the patient or family facing a possible endarterectomy should check the track record of both hospital and surgeon on this operation—and then, if necessary, simply seek help elsewhere. Your physician should be able to refer you to the nearest major center for such surgery. If he can't, you might try the chief teaching hospital of the nearest or largest medical school.

Dr. Hass suggests this as an alternative: "If surgical expertise is not available, or if our patient is very elderly and has a potentially serious medical problem which makes him a poor surgical risk, one should consider only those therapeutic strategies conventionally called medical treatment." And these, this expert points out, can be either of two kinds of medications: the anticoagulants or the antiplatelet drugs (such as aspirin).

Carotid endarterectomies are not the only operations today for TIAs and ischemic cerebrovascular disease such as occluded carotid arteries. A relatively new one is now being studied . . .

The New Cerebral Bypass Surgery

Although you may have heard of bypass surgery in connection with heart disease, you may well be hearing a lot more about it in connection with TIAs, strokes and other cerebrovascular diseases. It is the newest brain operation, but it utilizes one of the older cerebral surgical procedures. For this new bypass depends on the craniotomy technique perfected by Gigli in the last century.

In the mid-1960s, at the Medical College of Vermont, its professor of surgery, Dr. Raymond M. P. Donaghy, and the University of Zurich's professor of neurosurgery, Dr. M. Gazi Yasargil, worked together on experimental animals. They were testing a new operation. Beginning with a craniotomy to expose the brain, they used microsurgery to connect a scalp artery (the temporal) to a tiny segment of the middle cerebral artery on the surface of the brain. The plan was to supply blood to the brain of those with TIAs or with inoperable stenosis of the carotid or other vessels in the brain, or in those with mild or moderate ischemic strokes.

In late October 1967 Dr. Yasargil performed the first so-called extracranial-intracranial arterial bypass on a human patient in Zurich. By a strange coincidence, within twenty-four hours Dr. Donaghy performed the same operation on a patient in Vermont.

The operation—in terms of numbers performed—is a far cry from carotid endarterectomies; the most recent estimate made, in 1974, was that only 369 by-passes had been performed world-wide, with 163 of these in the United States. Probably all the bypasses done to date form only a small percentage of the number of endarterectomies done every month in the United States alone.

But bypasses are more delicate and trickier operations, besides being much newer and thus less well accepted. Those practicing this kind of surgery are, as is to be expected, enthusiastic about their successes. They feel it can revascularize the brain more successfully than the endarterectomies and that it can be used when the older operation cannot. NINCDS experts put their overview this way: "Far more important than the method selected for a cerebrovascular operation is the skill of the surgeon who performs it and his familiarity with the proposed technique. Bypass procedures may carry low mortality risk in the hands of one surgeon . . . whereas endarterectomy may be the method preferred by another." In fact, bypass surgery has even been performed on children.

Surgery for Hemorrhagic Stroke, Aneurysms and Malformations

Hemorrhagic strokes can occur as a result of hypertension which finally produces a break in a vessel. With prompt diagnosis (CT is especially valuable here), surgery may relieve the resultant neurological deficits by removing the blood clot (essentially a gel) pressing on the brain. The torn vessel can then be repaired, and the stroke symptoms gradually subside.

Aneurysms may be present even at birth but usually develop over the years in a weak spot in the arterial wall, often where an atherosclerotic plaque has caused damage. These blister- or sac-like formations may, as time passes, and particularly with hypertension, become thinned out just like a child's balloon that is blown up too much and finally bursts. Where possible, aneurysms are clipped (thanks to Harvey Cushing)—with metal clips that fasten at the sac's connection to the vessel wall. The blister may be surrounded with layers of fine muslin which prevent further leakage and cause dense scar tissue to form around the sac. Sometimes a sort of tissue glue—a chemical called cyanoacrylate—is painted on the sac, where it sticks and hardens to form a protective coating. Even silicon-iron mixtures have been injected into the sac and held there by a powerful magnet placed alongside the patient's head until the silicone jells to block off the aneurysm and prevent blood from getting into it again.

Sometimes the arteries and veins develop in a defective manner in one place, become enlarged and intertwined in a serpentine sort of way. This is called an angioma, or arteriovenous malformation. When it leaks blood or hemorrhages, the surgeon can sometimes removed it by locating each of the vessels leading into or away from the malformation and clipping these vessels one by one, then removing the structure (now sealed off from its blood supply). Sometimes such structures are simply cut off this way from the principal arteries filling them with blood, and then left untouched, since it may be too difficult to remove them safely. Sometimes it is even impossible to do so.

On occasion, small plastic spheres are injected into the carotid artery which act like so many emboli and block off the malformation's arteries. Other techniques too have been tried. In one, a tiny stainless-steel tip on a catheter is guided by powerful magnets to the formation. Once it is there, blood-clotting chemicals are sent through the catheter to fill the formation and make it a solid mass (virtually one well-contained blood clot) instead of blood-carrying vessels.

10

HOW STROKE VICTIMS CAN BE RETURNED TO LIFE

Recovery and Rehabilitation:
The Psychological Needs
and Problems of
Family and Victim;
the New Promise
for Long-Standing Paralysis

What You Must Know to Ensure
Help for Stroke

The facts are disturbing, even frightening. Of the 60 percent of the 600,000 Americans stricken with CVAs each year that do survive, virtually all initially suffer some degree of paralysis from their strokes. The latest NINCDS figures indicate that at least two thirds of these survivors are left with some degree of permanent disability, and many experts say that recovery is only rarely, if ever, complete. So our declining death rate from stroke is likely to be accompanied by an increase in the present 2.5 million disabled stroke survivors. There is greater hope today for stroke victims' recovery and rehabilitation then ever before—even for those who have suffered with their paralysis for two, three, five years and more. But what

of those stricken with massive strokes, what is the outlook for them
—paralyzed, with speech and perhaps vision and understanding,
memory and more all gone?

Modern rehabilitation along with the victim's will to health and
the family's support are the ingredients needed to produce modern
medical miracles. Take the experience and lesson of that lovely and
talented actress Patricia Neal. In her late thirties she suffered two
massive strokes in February 1965, with virtually all the concomitant damaging effects, from coma to paralysis to aphasia. Yet she
and her family refused to surrender and fought back resolutely
against the destructive effects of her illness. Despite all the damage
she suffered, this courageous woman was able to overcome all her
handicaps so steadily and effectively that she could make her first
public appearance in October 1966, less than two years after her
tragedy, when she was named Woman of the Year in London as
a token of the admiration and respect felt for her forthright struggle and in appreciation of her very inspiring example. In 1967 she
was able both to participate in the Motion Picture Academy
Awards and even to star in a film. Patricia Neal is proof of how
the human spirit can rise above catastrophe, and how, supported
by family, friends and medical expertise, a person can recover from
the terrible devastation of the most massive stroke to the point of
highest possible functioning.

We have also seen some of the tragedy of April Oursler Armstrong's stroke with its devastating aphasia and intellectual damage
to the young author and college professor. She had to literally start
from scratch, to learn to walk, talk, read, write, think, cook, laugh.
All the intellect and experiences of a lifetime had to be reassembled
into a functioning whole once more. Her book is a touching testi-
mony and a work of rare inspiration which can give those untouched by stroke a feeling for what it must be like to go through
the nightmare experience of CVA.

Such examples are the living proof of what Dr. Joseph Brudny,
New York University and ICD rehabilitation expert, insists should
be in the forefront of the minds of physicians, stroke victims and
their families: "The word 'never' should *never* cross our lips. The
positive attitude toward recovery must be present, we mustn't give

up." As this expert points out, he's not trying to say that everybody has the same hope of recovery—for example, should both sides of the brain be severely damaged, not enough brain tissue may be left to work with. But such a stroke—one affecting both sides—is, luckily, so rare that few physicians ever actually see one.

What You Should Know about Physical Medicine and Rehabilitation

It really began in World War II when forty-year-old Dr. Howard A. Rusk was commissioned a major and called to service in the Army Air Forces Medical Corps from his practice as an internist in St. Louis. Put in charge of two thousand convalescent young airmen, he was appalled by their treatment. After receiving the best possible medical and surgical care, they were totally neglected. Borrowing simple equipment, he got the men involved in doing things with their special skills, and this first rehabilitation effort paid off shortly in quicker recoveries and fewer relapses.

In charge of the entire Air Forces convalescent training division, and now a colonel, Rusk plunged into it with a program of physical therapy for both the bedridden and those already up and around. He involved these young men in their own treatment and therapy. Convalescence was cut 30 to 40 percent, and the young airmen were returned directly to combat units.

In 1943 he was put in charge of the centers for the severely wounded coming back from overseas—the amputees, the paraplegics, the blind, and the like. Rusk refused to just leave them in clean, well-cared-for wards where they would simply remain in physical comfort but social and psychological deterioration. Instead he devised programs of active physical and occupational therapy, educational retraining and psychological readjustment.

His successes convinced him of the value of this new approach for all medicine. So when Rusk left the Air Forces in 1945 he came to New York University to organize its department of physical medicine and rehabilitation, the first such comprehensive rehabilitation faculty at any medical school in the world. In 1948 he founded what is now officially known as the Institute of Rehabilitation Medicine, although many still refer to it as the Rusk Institute, and he still heads both the department and the institute.

His field is now a recognized specialty, and experts in this physical medicine and rehabilitation are known as physiatrists. They are certified as specialists in this field and they deal with the many problems which result in physical or mental disabilities. Their job is to put the whole thing together, to make it possible for the disabled person—the stroke victim, the paraplegic or quadriplegic, the arthritic—to function and live to the fullest extent that, with devices and training, his disabilities will permit. The physiatrist is the leader of the stroke rehabilitation team and should be found in charge of those facilities where stroke patients and others with disabilities are rehabilitated.

Dr. Rusk summarized his philosophy of rehabilitation medicine for me thus: "In a nutshell—taking the patient back to the best life possible. In our society, physical wholeness and ability are not synonymous—you can be the fastest runner or the highest jumper and yet be too stupid to make a living. We don't need many high jumpers and fast runners, so we pay for brains and hand skill primarily—that's the philosophy we've worked on since we developed this new concept of rehabilitation medicine."

Rehabilitation is actually a complex and dynamic process of total patient care. It should begin at the moment the acute-stroke victim is seen and diagnosed by the doctor, and every professional, paraprofessional and semiprofessional person who deals with this patient should be a part of the treatment process. It should not stop until the victim's best possible physical, psychological, social and vocational functioning has been reached. The underlying belief in this rehabilitation of the stroke patient is that every disabled human being has the right to the best therapies and techniques modern medicine has at its command—that the responsibility of medicine is to make it possible for this victim to again participate in his society to as far as his disorder and the damage it has done will allow. This process may be looked at from two aspects— recovery and rehabilitation.

Recovery from Stroke and Its Outlook

This is the healing process in the damaged brain itself that goes on after the acute stroke. As yet doctors can do little to influence this process beyond supporting the patient medically as best they can —by supplying oxygen, nutrients, comfort, and the like. Even the experts admit they cannot predict the outcome during the early days of a stroke. As Dr. James C. Folsom, director of ICD Rehabilitation and Research Center, explains from his extensive experience: "You don't know the first few days after a stroke—I've seen strokes that looked like they were going to be total disasters clear up and the individual become totally self-sufficient, while I've seen others that looked like they were going to be very minor and ended up being very devastating. Why, I don't know."

This mysterious natural healing process can—in the lucky ones —be so complete that it virtually clears up the entire problem by itself. Most stroke experts believe that this healing process in the injured brain is completed in a few weeks. Cerebral edema subsides during this time, and along with the recovery of the damaged nerve cells many of the difficulties may resolve themselves because the intracranial fluid pressure will no longer interfere with many brain functions. Nerve-cell healing may continue thereafter but experts feel that if the patient is not fully recovered by the end of the first month, he very likely will not do so later. But—a great deal of improvement can still take place and there is a vast amount of individual difference here. Most physicians in this field hesitate to make any definitive judgments on what the final natural recovery will be until at least six months after the stroke.

Here we must make a distinction between recovery and rehabilitation. The recovery is a natural healing process that is carried out by the cells and tissues of themselves with little opportunity for either victim or physician to influence this in any specific way. Perhaps the future will see new medical approaches which may offer ways of actually influencing this process in a positive fashion.

However—and this is the major point and chief distinction to be understood here—the victim can improve slowly but surely for a seemingly indefinite period thereafter. But this does require the untiring effort of patient and medical personnel alike, and no one really understands precisely how this improvement takes place, what things go on in the brain that permit such changes for the better to occur. This is the area of rehabilitation, of the deliberate effort to bring what is left to its maximum functioning level and to learn to compensate in little-understood ways for what has been lost.

We have some hints, however, of how this process works. For example, we discussed earlier how some nerve cells on the periphery of neural centers can take over that center's functioning under certain circumstances. As we shall also see shortly, rehabilitation people have now proved that improvement is possible many years after a stroke when seemingly a plateau of nonimprovement has been reached (and, traditionally, this plateau is considered to be six months).

When Does Rehabilitation Start?—What You Should Look For

If victim and family alike are not aware of the whole meaning of rehabilitation—when and where it should start, and how—a vital opportunity may be missed and the person destroyed by being condemned to a useless and terribly limited life quite unnecessarily. Knowing what care should be given, and how, is essential to protect yourself and your loved ones—for leaving a stroke victim severely disabled will likely cripple the family as well, and may destroy both.

First let us see what the experts advise for the rehabilitation of the stroke victim. As Dr. Folsom explains: "The rehabilitation process starts the minute of a stroke, and it's very important that the people in the health-care system have this attitude. The overriding factor is the expectation that the individual is going to keep working at it and that nobody's going to give up." Dr. Folsom urges that everyone talk to the patient while he is still unconscious even though no one really knows how much of this is heard and comprehended. Medical staff and family alike should simply talk to and reassure the patient, inform him of what has happened, where he is and what is being done for him, how his condition is, like: "Mr. Smith [or Daddy], you've had a stroke and you're in — — Hospital. Your pulse, heart and blood pressure are fine, we [the nurses, doctors] will be watching you constantly and turning you as needed. Everything will be taken care of and done to protect you . . . ," and so on.

An immediate evaluation from a physical-therapy point of view —the range of motion of stricken limbs and joints, sensory loss, and the like—is performed and continued regularly. The medical tests, care and medication we have already discussed. But the paralyzed leg and shoulder are placed and kept in proper position to prevent contracture and other muscle and joint problems later on. Passive motion or exercise of these limbs is carried out regularly by the nurses or physical therapist. As soon as the patient can begin to do such exercises with his good arm, he is taught to do so himself. As soon as the medical condition permits, he is brought to the physical- and occupational-therapy departments for active rehabilitation in which he can participate.

Dr. Folsom warns that "the biggest problem about stroke is the expectation that nothing can be done—but remarkable things are happening with stroke victims now, we're seeing people come back from strokes and be able to take care of themselves. The public needs to know how many people can and do recover from stroke." All those in the field recognize and emphasize the importance of motivation—of how much the victim and the family both desire a return to a functional life again.

It is possible for a person to have residual disabilities (weakness or poorly coordinated movements, say) without their affecting one's functioning. Such a person can return to his job, swim well and strongly, play tennis, do gymnastics. In fact, 90 percent of stroke victims will walk again, and 30 percent do return to work. But it is the upper limb, the arm, that is the most neglected part and therefore the one least often liable to recover. Now there is a exciting new hope for both the restoration of upper-limb use and an improvement in the use of the lower one as well.

According to NINCDS experts, "Undertreatment and overtreatment for stroke patients occur. The latter, which is less common, usually results from lack of knowledge, from anxiousness to please the patient or his family and, occasionally, from conscious economic abuse. Undertreatment is due most often to lack of knowledge or disinterest, unavailability of medical services and facilities." And Dr. Folsom warns stroke victims and families: "You ought to look out for overnursing—the worst thing you can do for people is to create dependency of one person on another."

New NINCDS cerebrovascular clinical research centers are being set up as focal points for work in prevention, diagnosis and therapy of stroke. Typically such units are staffed by as many as fifteen to twenty medical specialists, scientists, technicians and other personnel. But at the least, a stroke rehabilitation program should be available in every hospital where the stroke patient is to be treated, although the size and extent of these programs will vary widely. Your physician should be able to advise you on whether your local community hospital has such a program and whether it is adequate for your family member who suffers a stroke—but a discussion of this is certainly in order. Your doctor may in fact suggest moving the patient directly to a larger facility in a nearby community or he may do so after the immediate problem is under control and the patient can be safely transferred.

While large hospitals may have rehabilitation personnel who specialize in stroke, the smaller ones may have only a general-rehabilitation staff that works with all neurologically disabled patients and sometimes with all patients (as physical therapists may work with heart patients, arthritics, stroke victims, and so on). NINCDS experts suggest that certain specialists are needed for the successful rehabilitation of stroke patients, and you might check to see how many of these are available in the facility to which your doctor intends to send your family member.

The Stroke Rehabilitation Team

The core of any successful stroke-rehabilitation program is the rehabilitation team, those trained and experienced medical, paramedical and auxiliary people who function as a unit to make a combined effort to accomplish the complex ends sought in this field. To succeed, these professionals must be in constant consultation so that the input of each is considered in light of what the others are doing so that the team can evaluate what is being accomplished for the patient by the program, what can be done to improve his disabilities and to plan for further actions carefully individualized to bring this patient to his optimum functioning level. The personnel needed for a complete, sophisticated stroke team are:

1. **The family doctor:** His cooperation is essential and he should be available to contribute at staff conferences on his patient's improvement and the future plans for him.
2. **The neurologist:** This medical specialist determines the patient's neurological status, physical condition and capability as well as the prognosis.
3. **The physiatrist:** This expert's role is to evaluate the functional abilities and potentialities, to prescribe the rehabilitative therapy and to coordinate the team's activities.
4. **Other physicians:** Called in as needed may be neurological and vascular surgeons, ophthalmologist and psychiatrist, and many other medical specialists.
5. **General nurse:** Good nursing care saves lives in acute stroke, shortens recovery materially and protects patients from deformities by correct positioning in bed and handling.
6. **Rehabilitation nurse:** Ideally with special training in stroke; will make necessary referrals to other hospital resources, work with general nurses and with the family to prepare them and the patient for final discharge and home care.
7. **Physical therapist:** These are key team members to determine motor and sensory capacities and limitations, initiate therapeutic physical program to strengthen and help victim use limbs, walk better, and the like.
8. **Occupational therapist:** Analyzes complex overlapping problems such as speech, visual and sensory impairments; increases functional activities and self-care; teaches use of self-help devices

and advises on changes in home or office to facilitate more independent and extended activities of patient.

9. **Speech pathologist:** Evaluates communication problems, initiates speech therapy and advises family on how they can help.

10. **Social worker:** Assesses psychosocial needs, necessary home and community adaptations, economic situation; warns team of potential problems here—essential for adequate rehabilitation.

11. **Psychologist:** Does psychological evaluation and provides limited crisis therapy; determines any organic mental defects; helps with psychosocial (psychological and social) factors.

12. **Dietitian:** Ensures proper nutrition by planning a diet acceptable to the patient and in line with necessary medical restrictions.

13. **Vocational rehabilitation counselor:** Important in determining and helping with job rehabilitation or problems on the job.

Obviously only a large or specialized institution with a heavy patient load can afford to have these specialists available along with the sophisticated equipment and facilities that may be needed. Knowing the necessary rehabilitation personnel will give you the opportunity to evaluate the hospital your family member has been sent to. If it is a small community and far from a large city, it may be wise to consider transferral at an early stage to another facility for rehabilitation. But if the stroke is only a slight one, a good community hospital with an interested and knowledgeable family doctor, general physical-therapy facilities and a competent neurologist may be adequate for the task of rehabilitation.

A rehabilitation program—whether in a hospital stroke unit or a rehabilitation center such as Dr. Rusk's own institute—is not a custodial situation in which the patient is simply protected and cared for, where the victim has everything done for him. What can be accomplished does vary and must be approached realistically with the advice of experts, after adequate tests and examinations.

As Dr. Rusk explains: "We can rehabilitate these people because nature has such tremendous powers of compensation—some get back all they've lost, some a great deal, and some a fraction. It's our job to teach these people how to live the best life possible with what they have left. A program is prescribed for each individual —just like drugs or a diet. Patients work up to five hours a day at training until we get maximum improvement. The average training time for strokes is about seven weeks. Then they go back—to part-time or full-time employment, a new job; even a nursing home or custodial care, or whatever."

Help for the Emotional Needs of Stroke Victim and Family

The will-to-win, strong motivation, is the key to successful rehabilitation—the determination to recover and the feeling that it can be done. As Louis Pasteur said: "I have too much work unfinished." Dr. Folsom believes that the key to success here is to "get the individual to know what is going on, what you are trying to do and give him some sense of 'I can be a part of this process and I *can* get on top of this thing.' I can't stress this too strongly."

The family is surely the most important resource available to the stroke patient and his physician in every phase of rehabilitation. But the family needs help and support too—and this can come from essentially the same sources as those available to the patient. The whole stroke rehabilitation team is geared to helping the stroke victim both physically and psychologically, for it is well aware that the physical help will fail if the emotional is not there.

Psychological and psychiatric help are always near in a stroke unit. But for those in smaller communities it may be necessary to actually seek out this type of help, since a comprehensive stroke unit may not be available. Social workers are anxious to help victim and family in their readjustments to this changed and disturbed personal and family situation.

Our health-care system is comparatively effective in dealing with the physical disabilities produced by strokes, but there is a big gap left both by this system and by the medical profession in general in providing help for the psychosocial needs of our stroke victims and their families. Unless they actively seek such help, the recovery from stroke, in the sense of returning to a satisfying and good quality of life, will simply fail to be complete and leave much unhappiness in its wake.

Such help can be had from professionals in psychiatry, psychology and social work. Another comparatively new form of mental health help can be found in what is known as group therapy, which actually takes a number of forms. This help may be in the shape of the formal groups organized by many stroke and rehabilitation centers where the victims and/or their families (not just spouses and adult family members but sometimes even grandchildren) meet and talk about the experience and the problems of stroke. Here emotional support is obtained for those who have just suffered this problem and practical information is exchanged (such things as how to deal with common physical problems that arise, social ones and even financial tips). And then there are the immensely valuable Stroke Clubs, which help with the adjustments after the hospital's or rehabilitation center's work is done. In our next chapter we will suggest how you may go about finding some of these. The National Easter Seal can be of enormous help here.

Help for the Aphasias

This is a problem which crosses the line between the psychological and the neurological, for speech therapy partakes of both, plus a good deal all its own. Studies in the early 1970s have shown that the natural recovery process in the aphasias resulting from a stroke takes place within a three-month span. After that, any improvements are dependent on rehabilitation techniques.

Aphasia, as we have seen, is particularly frustrating to the patient. As the aphasic struggles to speak or make himself understood, to comprehend what he reads or hears, the frustration builds up until he finally explodes in an outburst of temper. Besides the anger, the loss of these basic powers produces depression and anxiety. Thus the aphasic sufferer needs a good deal of understanding and emotional support from those surrounding him and from the professionals who seek to rehabilitate him. Here, too, the psychologist and psychiatrist may prove invaluable. Yet those close to the aphasic—particularly spouses—repeatedly demonstrate an ability to communicate and to interpret what to the outsider or even the professional appears to be almost unintelligible speech.

Aphasia is one of the most highly individual aspects of stroke, with vast differences in degree and combinations of the various forms of communication affected. And just as individual as the disorder is, so must the therapy be. One family must know, for example, to approach the victim from the left side because he can no longer see the right side of his visual field.

Language therapy itself must be just as individual as the disorder itself and the results vary greatly. We have seen what can be accomplished by looking at the stories of Patricia Neal and April Armstrong—and how President Eisenhower's aphasia cleared spontaneously. Yet only recently has a Veterans Administration Cooperative Study provided documentary proof of the effectiveness of language therapy. This should in fact begin as soon as the stroke victim is sufficiently oriented and able to respond, because this treatment is thought to help spontaneous recovery and does reduce the anxiety in aphasic problems. Individually tailored therapy sessions are needed and their length is adjusted to the patient's fatigue level, varying from fifteen to sixty minutes, and scheduled once or twice a day. Group therapy, in addition, may also help because the social interaction in and of itself is of value.

The speech pathologist or therapist (the terms are used interchangeably) will use whatever means seem best and in whatever order. Some read better than they write or speak, or the other way around—the best form is emphasized first in therapy. In speech, most aphasics recover words in a particular order: nouns first, then verbs, adjectives, adverbs and then the rest. The speech therapists will work on words to be relearned in that same order—and will strive to first work with words that are particularly meaningful or important. Obviously "bed" or "eat" are more important for everyday use than "tape recorder" or "tango"—to pick some examples. Sometimes the words are even sung.

The family can help here immeasurably and the speech pathologist will explain just how. Some families in situations where such therapists were not available have even secured books and used them themselves to work with the patient's aphasia. A trained speech pathologist is of course preferable, but in aphasia, anything that works goes—and therapists are very flexible and use any methods themselves that seem most likely to help a particular aphasic.

Regaining the Use of Limbs— the Exciting New Hope

While it is true that 90 percent of stroke victims do learn to walk again, one must ask: How well do they walk? and What happens to the upper limb, to hand and arm? The answer to both has in the past been: Not good. One of the tragedies is that although all this can now be reversed, we're not doing enough about it! As Dr. Joseph Brudny explains: "If we had a Manhattan Project kind of approach to stroke, we would probably have half of the disabilities erased within a very brief period of time—half the stroke patients could return to a useful life!" Meanwhile, despite the numbers who learn to walk again, he points out: "Only 25 percent can regain the use of their arms because this was long neglected, since there was nothing to offer—now we do have something and this reverses the situation."

Normally when your hand or leg makes a move—in walking, picking up a glass, brushing your hair—innumerable muscles are involved. Some of these relax while the opposing ones contract to permit a highly complex and smoothly integrated action to take place. Normally, orders come down from your brain, and the "feedback"—the information from sensory nerve endings in your muscles—goes back to tell your brain that things are going according to long-established patterns while returning orders keep the muscles functioning until the entire movement has been carried out and completed.

In a stroke, however, this chain of command and the necessary feedback are disrupted as cerebral neurons and nerve tracts are interrupted, damaged or destroyed. Should this be a minor stroke with edema only temporarily disrupting communications, natural recovery restores the use of the limbs in a few weeks. Should the stroke be a major one, some damage will be permanent. But in stroke there is really not a true total paralysis as in the paraplegic, whose spinal cord is cut or broken. Instead the CVA victim suffers a spastic weakness or spastic paralysis.

In this spasticity the muscles are actually contracted, in spasm. They are very stiff and rigid, so that the limb resists any movement by the doctor or therapist. That is why the stroke victim so often has his wrist in a bent position with the fingers curled, on the affected side. This damaged brain simply cannot send out the proper messages—neither those ordering movements nor those ordering relaxation, nor can the feedback to say something is happening reach the appropriate healthy brain center. As a result of this lack of feedback, the limb "feels paralyzed." When the patient tries to walk, for example, the affected foot will drop from the ankle because he can't control or relax the spasms in the involved muscles that force the foot down, the stiff leg must be swung like a wooden limb, from the hip.

The conventional handling of these problems today is virtually to give up on the upper limb and to use braces or splints on the foot and lower limb, and a sling for the upper one. But along came Dr. Brudny and Dr. John V. Basmajian, professor of medicine at Canada's McMaster University, and others like them. They took the relatively new technique called biofeedback and turned it to use as a new hope of rehabilitation for stroke patients. As Dr. Basmajian puts it: "I think the time has come for us to recognize that a new revolution is in its beginning stages now, the revolution of behavioral medicine and biofeedback—the possibility that we can help human beings through their own resources and with the assistance of electronic gadgetry to compensate for deficiencies."

This Canadian expert points out that when physical therapists try to rehabilitate the upper limb in stroke victims, "the point achieved after several weeks or months of therapy is so dismal as to be almost worthless after the acute stage of stroke—in one study we found that only in about 3 or 4 percent of patients did aggressive physical therapy methods achieve any improvement worth all the trouble—but the same therapist using biofeedback techniques demonstrated that biofeedback in the upper limb is a very significant and useful therapy."

In this biofeedback technique, electrodes are placed on a chief muscle of the limb which has been useless to the stroke victim. When a muscle contracts or is used, a minute electrical current is generated. The electrodes pick up these tiny electrical signals and vastly magnify them to produce a display on what looks like a TV screen (such as is used in hospital monitoring of patients by electrocardiographs). Sometimes this magnified signal is used to produce a sound such as a beep as well. The screen display is commonly a white line, and both this and the sound vary with the degree to which the subject uses the muscle involved.

With the natural feedback system we all have (which tells us when a muscle is being used—in bending the wrist, say) we know when muscles are contracted or relaxed. But the stroke victim has lost this natural feedback system in his damaged brain. As a result he no longer has any way of knowing that the particular muscles are in spasm and cannot relax them. You can get some idea of all this by recalling how when your hand falls asleep and you try to do something with it, you fail—without this feedback information from your muscles you can't turn a lamp on or write until the feeling comes back.

With this new feedback technique the stroke victim can see or hear that his muscles are responding to his commands to them—actual proof that he can command these muscles in some way. As he strives to make them obey more he can relearn how to gain some control over the particular muscle he is working on by using the information from the machine—the sound or signal tells him the muscle is reacting as he strives either to move the hand, say, or to relax the muscle so his wrist uncurls and is usable. Once the spasm is relaxed he can start to use the muscle, for the limb is no longer rigid. While the pre-stroke normal use and control will not return, the stroke victim can slowly make his "paralyzed" limb functional once more and learn to use it for the various purposes he may desire.

Dr. Brudny likes to term this "sensory feedback" because the machine is taking the place of the neural feedback that has been

lost. And it does work as the victim struggles to better his perform-
ance in each session—to make the white line rise higher or the
sound louder. Slowly the spasms are relaxed, the muscle is able to
be used more. Exactly how this change occurs in the brain is not
understood yet and it does take months and even years, but it can
and does happen if the person works at it both at home and with
the therapist.

Stroke victims are astounded to discover that even several years
after their stroke and after being told "It's six months since your
stroke and you still can't use your limb, so just forget it,"—they
can now use that same limb. The wrist and fingers can be relaxed,
the foot raised and the leg used in walking rather than being
dragged along like a stiff piece of wood. With the steady encourage-
ment of the doctor, and hard work and determination on the part
of the patient, weakened and unused limbs are brought slowly back
to a point where they can actually serve some functional use, where
they can be of real help and benefit to the sufferer in his everyday
life. Arms need no longer be carried useless in a sling; leg braces
and splints need no longer be worn, while the gait improves and
quickens.

There is proof that stroke victims several years after their CVAs,
after being given up by conventional rehabilitation techniques can
be successfully retrained in the use of limbs. Dr. Brudny and his
team have found that 60 percent of stroke sufferers, a year or more
after their CVAs and after being given up by those in conventional
rehabilitation, can improve the use of their affected limbs with
biofeedback. This is being confirmed by others elsewhere in the
United States and in Canada. Dr. Brudny sets an eight-week trial
period after which those who fail to show improvement must, he
feels, be given up.

So while this biofeedback is not the ultimate panacea, it does
promise hope to the majority of stroke victims with useless limbs,
and the upper limbs in particular, since these are so rarely helped
by conventional therapy today. This biofeedback technique is
spreading so rapidly that if you want to try it, your doctor is likely
to know of some center in your area where it is being used or at
least being tried.

Obviously the entire or even the final answers are still a long way off, but NINCDS experts see the picture this way: "Stroke is viewed by many as the most devastating and disabling of all human disorders. If the momentum of research can be sustained, the promise for improving the quality of life everywhere can be fulfilled." The future is surely brighter than the past—and our next and last chapter will give you some sources of information and help which may be of particular use to you should you or someone in your family suffer this tragic disorder.

11

SOURCES OF HELP AND INFORMATION FOR STROKE VICTIMS AND THEIR FAMILIES

With the growing interest and involvement of physicians and medical scientists in stroke, there is a burgeoning volume of knowledge which promises many changes in the coming years. Victims and their families often have special needs and desire certain kinds of information for their problems, or want simply to keep up with the advances that certainly lie ahead. Here are the sources of such information (along with their addresses) to which you can turn. These are divided into the following sections for your convenience:

1. General overall information on stroke—organizations that are specifically interested in CVAs in all their aspects
2. Atherosclerosis and diet
3. Hypertension and exercise
4. Rehabilitation, aphasia and psychological problems
5. Stroke clubs

1. For General Information: Here, alphabetically, are the organizations which are interested in cerebrovascular diseases in all their aspects.

American Heart Association
7320 Greenville Avenue
Dallas, Tex. 75231

AHA is involved and concerned with just about every aspect of cardiovascular disease including stroke, hypertension, atherosclerosis, and the rest. It publishes an unequaled variety of pamphlets and informational materials which you can obtain from your local chapter. However, should you live in a tiny community or rural area with no chapter available, you can write the national center above for materials on those aspects of stroke in which you are interested. The information is of course authoritative, for AHA has a vast array of experts working with it and publishes numerous scientific journals (such as the medical journal *Stroke*) and holds regular medical conferences for the professions. AHA depends on voluntary contributions to make its important and continuing work possible.

American Medical Association
535 North Dearborn Street
Chicago, Ill. 60610

AMA has an ever-growing number of pamphlets on various aspects of health. A note will bring you a list of these, and you can choose among them. Currently, for example, there are booklets on exercise, losing weight and hypertension.

National Easter Seal Society
2023 West Ogden Avenue
Chicago, Ill. 60612

Easter Seal is unique in that it is strictly a service organization with local societies across the country providing a whole range of rehabilitation services for stroke victims, along with innovative new programs in various aspects of this. In addition, Easter Seal has a large variety of booklets and educational materials covering every aspect of stroke rehabilitation, including aphasia. This organization is, in fact, the largest not-for-profit provider of stroke services in the United States. Its aim is to serve the handicapped in general, and publications are available at state and local societies, or if none are available where you live, then through the national office above. Easter Seal depends on voluntary contributions to make its important and continuing work possible.

National Heart, Lung, and Blood Institute
9000 Rockville Pike
Bethesda, Md. 20205

NHLBI is concerned with the aspects of the cardiovascular problems in its name. Its Information Office can supply materials on stroke, atherosclerosis, hypertension and diet. Its volume of *Arteriosclerosis* has become a medical classic, but it is technical. However, its *Fact Sheet on Arteriosclerosis* is available and useful. NHLBI has done a splendid job in its field, for the public and medical profession alike.

National High Blood Pressure Education Program
National Institutes of Health
120/80 NIH
Bethesda, Md. 20205

NHBPEP is just what its name says—an education program designed to make information on hypertension available to the public. A vast amount can be obtained by writing to its Information Office.

National Institute of Neurological and Communicative
  Diseases and Stroke
9000 Rockville Pike
Bethesda, Md. 20205

NINCDS is deeply interested in stroke in all its forms and aspects (from causes to diagnosis, therapy to rehabilitation). It is involved in backing stroke units and research, is concerned with the aphasias and communication problems. Actually, there is no aspect of stroke that does not concern NINCDS, and a letter to its Information Office will bring a good deal of helpful information— its clinical, epidemiological and clinical aspects. NINCDS's publication, *Fundamentals of Stroke Care,* is surely a medical classic in the field, although it is technical and runs to nearly five hundred pages. One must compliment NINCDS for the magnificent job it has done, serving both the public and medical profession alike.

2. Atherosclerosis and Diet: Both NINCDS and NHLBI are very much interested in these problems and have materials available. NHLBI also has diets for various medical problems.

AHA, too, has informational material on atherosclerosis. The new edition of the *American Heart Association Cookbook* is of value for low-cholesterol diets.

The AMA also has pamphlets on reducing and diets available.

3. Hypertension and Exercise: All the organizations listed under 1. are interested in these problems and can offer information on them. Then there are the following for exercise information:

President's Council on Physical Fitness and Sports
400 Sixth Street, S.W.
Washington, D.C. 20201

American Alliance for Health, Physical Education and Recreation
1201 16th Street, N.W.
Washington, D.C. 20036

4. Rehabilitation, Aphasia and Psychological Problems: Easter Seal's whole program is geared to rehabilitation, so that it has active service programs in these areas and very considerable amounts of literature available on every aspect of all three of these problems which are so very closely related. NINCDS is very interested in aphasia and the related communication problems.

AHA, too, has some excellent material and two outstanding booklets: *Strike Back at Stroke,* which shows how the family can arrange the bed and exercise the stroke victim, and it gives self-exercises as well; and *Do It Yourself Again* is an invaluable booklet of self-help devices to make the stroke victim independent (everything from special knives and food plates to wheelchairs, devices for writing, sewing, cooking, dressing, household chores).

Should you or your physicians seek a qualified rehabilitation facility (or check on one) in your area, you can contact the organization which accredits, certifies and lists these along with their addresses and the names of the qualified people directing them:

National Association of Rehabilitation Facilities
5530 Wisconsin Avenue, N.W.
Washington, D.C. 20015

And for the names of specialized personnel in your area:

Speech pathologists
American Speech and Hearing Association
10801 Rockville Pike
Rockville, Md. 20852

Physical therapists
American Physical Therapy Association
1156 15th Street, N.W.
Washington, D.C. 20005

Occupational therapists
American Occupational Therapy Association
6000 Executive Boulevard
Rockville, Md. 20852

5. *Stroke Clubs:* Both AHA and Easter Seal have extensive lists of stroke clubs available for the asking which may be of help to you. Moreover, your local Easter Seal Society will even work with you to set up a stroke club in your community if there is a need for one but none yet available.

Where stroke is concerned, the past has been a gloomy picture in every way. But the future promises hope in the things that really matter: prevention, treatment, even cure, and rehabilitation.

BIBLIOGRAPHY

To record here all the hundred and more references (medical and other professional articles, textbooks and monographs) would actually be counterproductive, for most readers would find so extensive a bibliography only a hindrance to locating those readily obtainable and understandable sources of specific in-depth information on their particular interest. Here, then, are a limited number of such references, chosen for being of the greatest value to the largest number of readers while simultaneously demanding the least technical knowledge:

Armstrong, A. O., *Cry Babel.* New York, Doubleday, 1979.

Barnett, H. J. M., *et al.,* "Aspirin—Effective in Males Threatened with Stroke." *Stroke* (July-August 1978).

Brown, M., and Glassenberg, M., "Mortality Factors in Patients with Acute Stroke." *Journal of the American Medical Association* (June 11, 1973).

Brudny, J., *et al.,* "Helping Hemiparetics to Help Themselves." *Journal of the American Medical Association* (February 23, 1979).

———, "Sensory Feedback Therapy for Stroke Patients." *Geriatrics* (June 1976).

Collaborative Group for the Study of Stroke in Young Women, "Oral Contraception and Increased Risk of Cerebral Ischemia or Thrombosis." *New England Journal of Medicine* (April 26, 1973).

———, "Oral Contraceptives and Stroke in Young Women." *Journal of the American Medical Association* (February 17, 1975).

"Conquering Strokes Depends on Timely Treatment." *MGH News* (June–August, 1976).

Crick, F. H. C., "Thinking About the Brain." *Scientific American* (September 1979).

Crickmay, M. C., *Help the Stroke Patient to Talk.* Springfield, Thomas, 1976.

Dubos, R. J., *Louis Pasteur, Free Lance of Science.* New York, Scribners, 1976.

Dyken, M. L., *et al.,* "Cooperative Study of Hospital Frequency and Character of Transient Ischemic Attacks." *Journal of the American Medical Association* (February 28, 1977).

Evarts, E. V., "Brain Mechanisms of Movement." *Scientific American* (September 1979).

Freese, A. S.: *You and Your Hearing.* New York, Scribners, 1980.

———, *The Miracle of Vision.* New York, Harper & Row, 1977.

Garroway, W. M., Whisnant, J. P., *et al.,* "The Declining Incidence of Stroke." *New England Journal of Medicine* (March 1, 1979).

Geschwind, N., "Language, Aphasia, and Related Disorders," in *Textbook of Medicine,* by Beeson and McDermott, 14th ed., Philadelphia, Saunders, 1970.

———, "Specialization of the Human Brain." *Scientific American* (September 1979).

Golden, G. S., "Strokes in Children and Adolescents." *Stroke* (March–April 1978).

Goldstone, J., and Moore, W. S., "A New Look at Emergency Carotid Artery Operation . . ." *Stroke* (November–December 1978).

Gresham, G. F., *et al.,* "Residual Disability in Survivors of Stroke —the Framingham Study." *New England Journal of Medicine* (November 6, 1975).

Hockett, C. F., *Man's Place in Nature.* New York, McGraw-Hill, 1973.

Hubel, D. H., "The Brain." *Scientific American* (September 1979).

Hutchinson, E. C., and Acheson, E. J., *Strokes (Natural History, Pathology and Surgical Treatment).* London, Saunders, 1975.

Kannel, W. B., "Recent Findings from the Framingham Study." *Medical Times* (April 1978).

Kety, S. S., "Disorders of the Human Brain." *Scientific American* (September 1979).

Levy, R. I., "Stroke Decline, Implications and Prospects." *New England Journal of Medicine* (March 1, 1979).

McDowell, F. H., "Cerebrovascular Diseases," in *Textbook of Medicine,* by Beeson and McDermott. 14th ed. Philadelphia, Saunders, 1970.

Millikan, C. H., and McDowell, F. H., "Treatment of Transient Ischemic Attacks." *Stroke* (July–August 1978).

National Heart, Lung, and Blood Institute, *Arteriosclerosis Fact Sheet.* U.S. Government Printing Office, 1978.

Nauta, W. J. H., and Feirtag, M., "The Organization of the Brain." *Scientific American* (September 1979).

Page, I. H., "Two Cheers for Hypertension." *Journal of the American Medical Association* (December 7, 1979).

Petitti, D.B., *et al.:* "Risk of Vascular Disease in Women." *Journal of the American Medical Association* (September 14, 1979).

Pool, J. L., *Your Brain and Nerves.* New York, Scribners, 1978.

Reinmuth, O. M., "Intracranial Bypass Surgery for Cerebral Arterial Disease." *Stroke* (January–February 1979).

———, "Prologue," in *Fundamentals of Stroke Care.* Ed. by A. L. Sahs and E. C. Hartman. U.S. Department of Health, Education and Welfare, 1976.

Report by the Comptroller General of the United States, *Recommended Dietary Allowances.* Washington, D.C., U.S. General Accounting Office, November 30, 1978.

Sahs, A. L.; Hartman, E. C., and Aronson, S. M. (eds.), *Guidelines for Stroke Care.* Washington, D.C., U.S. Department of Health, Education and Welfare, 1976.

"Salt and High Blood Pressure." *Consumer Reports* (March 1979).

Soltero, I., "Trends in Mortality from Cerebrovascular Diseases in the United States, 1960 to 1975." *Stroke* (November–December 1978).

Stevens, C. F., "The Neuron." *Scientific American* (September 1979).

Taylor, M. L., *Understanding Aphasia.* New York, The Institute
of Rehabilitation Medicine, N.Y.U. Medical Center, 1970.

Toole, J. F., "Can an Aspirin a Day Keep a Stroke Away?" *Executive Health* (January 1979).

INDEX

About the Author

ARTHUR S. FREESE is a full-time free-lance writer specializing in medicine, psychiatry and related areas. He is the author or co-author of over twenty books, including *You and Your Hearing; The End of Senility; Help for Your Grief;* and *Low Back Pain.* Contributing editor to *Modern Maturity* magazine, Freese has written for over seventy magazines, including *Saturday Review, Good Housekeeping, Better Homes & Gardens* and *Ladies' Home Journal.*